Defeat COMMON COLD AND NOSE ALLERGIES

Includes:
- Homeopathy • Biochemics • Bach Flower Remedies
- Nasal Irrigation • Yoga • Ayurveda • Naturopathy
- TCM • Nutritional Supplements

Dr. Harilakshmi Jayachandran

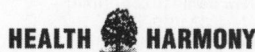

HEALTH HARMONY
An imprint of
B. Jain Publishers (P) Ltd.
USA — Europe — India

DEFEAT COMMON COLD AND NOSE ALLERGIES

First Edition: 2009
2nd Impression: 2013

All rights reserved. No part of this book may be reproduced, stored in a retrieval system or transmitted, in any form or by any means, mechanical, photocopying, recording or otherwise, without any prior written permission of the author.

© with the publisher

Published by Kuldeep Jain for
HEALTH HARMONY
An imprint of
B. Jain Publishers (P) Ltd.
1921/10, Chuna Mandi, Paharganj, New Delhi 110 055 (INDIA)
Tel.: +91-11-4567 1000 • Fax: +91-11-4567 1010
Email: info@bjain.com • Website: www.bjain.com

Printed in India by
J.J. Offset Printers

ISBN: 978-81-319-0675-0

"The mind is a fire to be kindled, not a verset to be filled."

Platarch (66 AD)

Publisher's Note

Respiratory infections and allergies worldwide continue to be major cause of morbidity both for children as well as adults. Careless prescription of antibiotics and antiallergics at random are only accounting for repeated incidences as the attack is not directed at the root level. With Homeopathy and other alternative therapies fast becoming popular, people today have more options to choose from and tackle their problems as effectively as ever.

With 'Defeat Common Cold and Nose Allergies', our objective is to educate the masses on the therapeutic benefits of Homeopathy, Ayurveda, Naturopathy, Yoga, TCM, Bach flower therapy etc. in recurring colds and nasal allergies. Care has been taken to include a detailed clinical background of these with a systematic proposition of the most commonly indicated remedies under each speciality. Some useful illustrations on the various yogic asanas have been included for practical purposes.

We hope that this work will provide all the information that one needs to know on effective management of colds in general and will be equally useful for the layperson as well as the sophisticated practitioner.

Kuldeep Jain
CEO, B.Jain Publishers

Acknowledgement

This work is dedicated with silent gratitude to Dr. Rangachari who is a constant source of inspiration and encouragement to all his students.

I wish to thank all the past and present teachers in our school for their patient understanding and guidance. My special thanks to Mrs. Malathi Raghava (truly a friend, guide and philosopher) for kindling my interest in this fascinating field.

I would also like to express my sincere thanks and appreciation to all my classmates and friends. It has been an interesting and enjoyable experience to explore and learn homeopathy in their cheerful and interactive companionship.

I very much appreciate the moral support given by my better half, Jaya, during this new venture into healing through homeopathy.

Preface

The inspiration to take up thesis on Common Cold and Nose Allergies came from observation of several cases with these problems in free clinics run by Dr. Rangachari in Singapore. The patients were frustrated since they could not carry out their daily chores due to sneezing episodes with running nose. They were also greatly concerned about being heavily dependent on anti-histamines almost on a daily basis. As no specific allergen could be identified and therefore the cause of symptoms could not be determined. Research of literature showed that the conventional treatment does not afford much relief to these patients. These cases are now being treated homeopathically with satisfactory results. There has been a dramatic decrease in patients' dependence on anti-histamines and the symptoms are manageable by homeopathic means alone.

From homeopathic concept, treatment would be decided by the symptoms alone which are very similar for the various types of rhinitis, whether allergic or non-allergic in origin. In this thesis, a coherent picture of *recurrent colds* has been presented discussing its pathology and symptomatology, and finally its management by means of homeopathic treatment. Other holistic therapies which are helpful have also been mentioned. Allergic rhinitis has been included and discussed where necessary for comparison.

Contents

Publisher's Note v
Acknowledgement vi
Preface ix

1. Introduction 1
2. Anatomy of Nose and it's Functions 5
3. Rhinitis – Definition and Symptomatology 7
4. Rhinitis – Classification at a Glance 9
5. Allergic Rhinitis - Types, Description and Clinical Features 10
6. Non-allergic Rhinitis - Types, Description and Clinical Features 13
7. Etiology of Chronic Non-allergic Idiopathic Rhinitis .. 21
8. Pathophysiology of Non-allergic/idiopathic Rhinitis ... 27
9. Mechanisms Operating in different forms of Non-allergic Rhinitis 33
10. Complications of Persistent or Recurring Rhinitis 36
11. Non-allergic Rhinitis in Special Cases 38
12. Diagnostic Tests 42
13. Differential Diagnosis 46
14. Lifestyle and Management Advice to Rhinitis Patients 49

15. Conventional Treatment of Non-allergic Rhinitis and its Drawbacks 53
16. Homeopathic Perspective of Non-allergic Rhinitis 58
17. Homeopathic Remedies from different groups – A look at the repertories 61
18. Treatment of Recurring Allergic / Non allergic Rhinities – A miasmatic approach 69
19. Important Remedy Profiles in Rhinitis Treatment I - Acute Remedies 76
20. Important Remedy Profiles in Rhinitis Treatment II - Deep Acting Remedies 97
21. Homeopathic Management of Non-allergic Rhinitis- A Case Analysis 113
22. Some interesting case studies in brief 123
23. Supplementary therapies – Biochemic salts and Bach flower remedies 129
24. Alternative Methods – A Holistic Approach 136
25. Nasal Wash and Nasal Sprays 139
26. Yoga Therapy 141
27. Ayurveda 156
28. Naturopathy Combined with Yoga 162
29. TCM – Traditional Chinese Medicine 164
30. Nutritional Supplements and Dietary Advice to Patients 169
31. Conclusion – Living with Rhinitis 175
    Bibliography 177
    Appendix – A general questionnaire designed for rhinitis patients 179

CHAPTER 1

Introduction

RHINITIS

Rhinitis affects millions of people all over the world and results in significant symptomatology. Rhinitis is inflammation of the inner lining of the nose and may be characterized by an itchy/running nose, sneezing, and nasal congestion. The exact classification of rhinitis has long been debated in the literature. In 1999, the World Health Organization introduced a new classification[1] for *Allergic Rhinitis (ARIA Guidelines)*[1], *dividing* in into two categories: Intermittent Allergic Rhinitis and a Persistent Allergic Rhinitis.

However, *Rhinitis* may now be generally divided into two basic types: *Allergic and Non-allergic. Although, the symptoms of allergic and non-allergic rhinitis overlap significantly, but the causes appear to be entirely different.* Whatever be the mechanism, the various rhinitis syndromes result in significant morbidity, affecting the quality of work and life of the population in all countries.

Non-allergic rhinitis/Common cold

In recent years, there has been an increasing incidence of recurrent cold not caused by any allergen. Although patients show typical symptoms of nasal allergy, all diagnostic techniques to detect allergic response proves negative. These patients are said to suffer from *chronic or recurrent non-allergic rhinitis* (also known as *idiopathic rhinitis,* since the cause is often unknown). They are treated by conventional medicine in a fashion similar to allergic rhinitis (hay fever), using the *ARIA Guidelines*

Some patients have many symptoms with eosinophils present in their nasal discharge and this condition is termed a Non-Allergic Rhinitis with Eosinophilia Syndrome (NARES). Other examples of non-allergic rhinitis are:

i. hormonal rhinitis ii. vasomotor rhinitis iii. occupational rhinitis iv. gustato rhinitis v. drug-induced rhinitis.

These forms of chronic, non-infectious rhinitis represent a spectrum of nasal disorders that are best categorized as a *hyper-reactive of the nasal mucosa to a variety of stimuli.*

What happens in non-allergic rhinitis?

Nasal hypersensitivity occurs when *non-allergic irritants* such as perfume, tobacco smoke, ozone, sulphur dioxide, nitrogen dioxide, cold air and other environmental pollutants result in irritational nasal membrane and increased leakiness, increased nerve excitability and infilteration of white blood cell and mast cells in the superficial nasal membranes. These factors lead to *increased nasal irritability.* Few old blood pressure medications such as reserpine, methyldopa, ACE inhibitors and alpha blockers as well as Hormone Replacement Therapy (HRT) may also cause nasal obstruction. The last trimester of pregnancy is also associated with worsening of symptoms due to hormonal factors.

Increasing incidence

Over the last 30 years, the prevalence of chronic rhinitis has been increasing. It is estimated[2] that more than 10% of the population in the U.S. alone has chronic or recurrent nasal obstruction, congestion, rhinorrhea, sneezing and pruritus. Approximately half the number of these patients are classified having chronic allergic and other half as having chronic non-allergic rhinitis, including vasomotor rhinitis. *The National Classification Task Force* in the U.S. has recently concluded that at least *17 million Americans have non-allergic rhinitis.*

Keeping in view the protiferation of all kinds of medication amongst general public ever increasing pollution, *it is not surprising that the incidence of non-allergic rhinitis is on rise.* Other contributing factors include the stressfull life style in addition to the occupational and environmental hazards that were non-existent until the last century. *One prime example is the extensive use of air-conditioners in home and office, especially* in countries with a hot climate. Exposure to cold and dry air inside the room alternating with hot air outside, contributes a lot towards conditions favoring chronic rhinitis.

Health-economic factors

The adverse effect that recurrent rhinitis has on patients health and resources is quite substantial. There are an ever increasing number of visits to doctor. It has been reported by the *Agency for Healthcare Research and Quality (AHRQ)*[3] that the treatment costs for rhinitis runs into billions of dollars, in the United States alone. The annual direct cost to the economy is enormous due to treatment and medication expenses, as well as loss of productivity to employers and society.

Demand for holistic therapy

Conventional treatment, so far, has been empirical and not really satisfactory. It has been acknowledged that traditional anti-histamines and the newer less-sedating antihistamines have no established benefit in the treatment of non-allergic rhinitis. Medications such as systemic sympathomimetic amines relieve symptoms but are not recommended for regular long-term use. Topical vasoconstrictors should be avoided because they cause the vasculature of the nasal mucous membrane to lose its sensitivity to other vasoconstrictive stimuli, for e.g. the humidity and temperature of inspired air. Moreover, their administration delays proper treatment while incurring significant cost and burden to the health care system.

Hence *a new trend is emerging towards a more holistic approach* and there is a growing demand by the general public for alternative therapies in preference to conventional medication. A holistic approach to the problem is likely to yield better results. Management by holistic therapy, naturally includes alternative as well as supportive methods which include yoga exercises and breathing techniques.

Treatment by homeopathy

This book was written by observing *recurrent cases of common cold*. The patients were given acute remedies to relieve the symptoms whenever necessary and this was followed by long term miasmatic treatment in each. These patients have shown very good improvement after starting homeopathic treatment, with dramatic decline in their dependence on anti-histamines.

REFERENCES

1. http://www.allergy-clinic.co.uk/hayfever.htm
2. http://www.allergyhealthcare.com/article%2013.htm
3. http://www.aafp.org/sfp/20050915/1057.html

Chapter 2

Anatomy of Nose and It's Functions

The purpose of the nose is to warm, clean and humidify the air that is inspired. In addition, it helps in smelling and tasting. *A normal person will produce about two quarts of fluid (mucus) each day* which aids in keeping the respiratory tract clean and moist. Tiny microscopic hair (cilia) line the surface helping to brush away particles. Eventually this mucus blanket is moved to the back of the throat where it is unconsciously swallowed. This entire process in closely regulated by several body systems.

NASAL SEPTUM

The nose is divided into two passages by cartilage which is called as the septum. Protruding into each breathing passage are bony projections, called turbinates, which help to increase the inner surface area of nose. There are three turbinates on each side of the nose (inferior, middle and superior). The sinuses are four paired air filled chambers which empty into the nasal cavity. The purpose of sinuses is to keep the skull light in weight.

ROLE OF MUCUS

The nasal passages are lined with a membrane that produces mucus. Mucus is one of the body's defence systems and if it has following set of functions:

- Mucus is a clear liquid which traps small particles and bacteria that are drawn into the nose as the person inhales.

- The trapped bacteria usually remain harmless in healthy individuals.

In non-allergic rhinitis, there appears to be an imbalance in the function of nerves that make mucus glands secrete fluid and which causes blood vessels to swell or contract. Common complaints are blockage, runny nose, post-nasal drip along with sneezing and itching. The condition usually lasts for years.

Post-nasal Discharge

Post-nasal discharge is a mucus accumulation in the back of the nose and throat leading to or giving the sensation of mucus dripping downward from the back of the nose. Chronic rhinitis is characterized by persistent irritation and inflammation of the lining tissues of the nose. One of the most common characteristics of chronic rhinitis is post-nasal drip. Post-nasal drip may lead to chronic sore throat. Post-nasal drip can be caused by excessive thick secretions or an impairment in the normal clearance of mucus from the nose and throat.

Nasal Drainage and an Abnormal Production of Nasal Secretions

A number of factors result in an increase or decrease in nasal drainage. Increase in thin secretions may result from cold temperatures, spicy food or medication. *Thickened secretions* can be the result of environmental irritants or nasal infections.

REFERENCES

1. http://www.umm.edu/patiented/articles/what_rhinitis_000077_1.htm
2. http://www.emedicine.con/ent/topic402.htm
3. http://www.medicinenet.com/chronic_rhinitis/page2.htm
4. http://www.ncbi.nlm.nih.gov/entrez/query
5. http://www.gpnotebook.co.uk/simplepage.cfm?ID=-1147535310&linkID=29880&cook=yes

CHAPTER 3

Rhinitis - Definition and Symptomatology

DEFINITION

Rhinitis is inflammation of the nasal mucous membrane which may be caused by allergic irritants or other factors.

Allergic Rhinitis

Rhinitis is allergic reaction of the nasal mucosa occurring in response to allergen seasonally (hay fever) or perennially.

Non-allergic Rhinitis

Rhinitis due to non-allergic stimuli such as irritants, chilling anger, etc. It is also known as *'idiopathic rhinitis'* when it occurs without a known cause.

COMMON SYMPTOMS
• Running nose
• Sneezing
• Stuffy nose and nasal congestion
• Itching in nose or mouth
• Congested and watering eyes
• Ears feel blocked
• Sticking sensation in throat
• Headache and fatigue

COMMONLY USED TERMINOLOGY

Acute Rhinitis: Inflammation of the nose that occurs for only a few days. Typically this is caused by a virus if it goes on beyond a week, then it is probably bacterial. Same as common cold.

Allergens: Normally harmless substances which produces an exaggerated *allergic reaction* inflammatory response in sensitive idiosyncratic people.

Allergic Rhinitis: It is an immune response to allergans. Medical term for hay fever, a condition due to allergy *that mimics a chronic cold*. (Hay fever is a misnomer since hay is not a usual cause of this problem and there is no fever). Many substances cause these allergic symptoms in hay fever. Allergic rhinitis is the correct term for this allergic reaction. (Rhinitis means "irritation of the nose" and is a derivative of Rhino, meaning "nose.")

Chronic Rhinitis: Inflammation of the nose that goes on from weeks to months, which is different from "cold" and may be caused by allergy, nasal irritants, structural, or physiological problems.

Non-allergic Rhinitis: Inflammatory condition of the nose without an obvious allergic cause.

Vasomotor Rhinitis: A type of non-allergic rhinitis, by an abnormal neuronal control of the blood vessels supplying the nose. Also known as *idiopathic rhinitis.*

Nasal Irritants: Nasal irritants usually do not lead to the typical response seen with classical allergies, but they can mimic or make allergies worse. Examples of these irritants include cigarette smoke, perfume, aerosol sprays, smoke and car exhaust.

Post-nasal Drip: Mucus accumulation in the back of the nose leading to the sensation of mucus dripping downward from the back of the nose.

CHAPTER 4

Rhinitis – Classification at a Glance

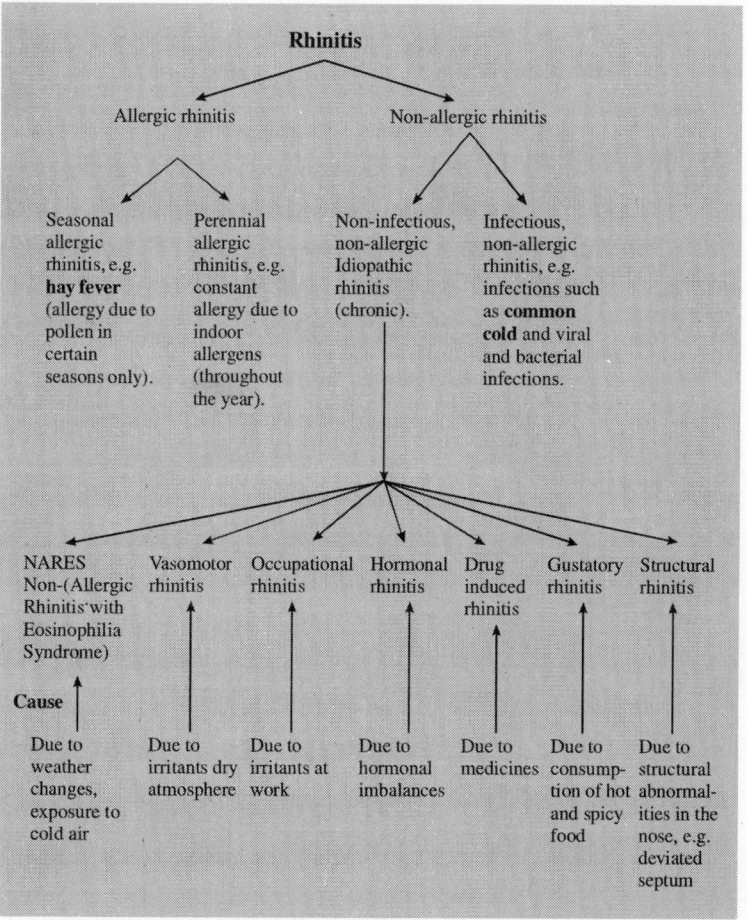

CHAPTER 5

Allergic Rhinitis – Types, Description and Clinical Features

As earlier seen the classification chart, the two basic types of rhinitis are: *allergic rhinitis and non-allergic rhinitis*. In order to understand non-allergic rhinitis which is the topic of this thesis, *it is useful to first know the features of allergic rhinitis.*

ALLERGIC RHINITIS

Allergic rhinitis is diagnosed when *specific antigens can be identified* and is often sub-classified as:

1. Seasonal allergic rhinitis (Hay fever)
2. Perennial allergic rhinitis

A new classification was introduced by the World Health Organization in the year 1999, for allergic rhinitis (*ARIA Guidelines*). The purpose was to try and create similar treatment guidelines for asthma and allergic rhinitis which often co-exist in the same patient (80% of asthma sufferers have concomitant allergic rhinitis).

Instead of the traditional seasonal and perennial divisions, W.H.O. introduced *Intermittent Allergic Rhinitis* and *Persistent Allergic Rhinitis*. Intermittent would replace the seasonal (hay fever) type disease and persistent would replace perennial rhinitis (but some overlap does take place). These two groups are then further sub-divided into *Mild, Moderate and Severe* symptoms and treated according to the new guidelines.

Seasonal Allergic Rhinitis

The most common type of allergic rhinitis is the seasonal allergic rhinitis such as *hay fever*, which has been reported to affect more than 20% of the U.S. population. Airborne pollens from grass, tree and weeds serve as the causes of seasonal allergic rhinitis. Seasonal allergic rhinitis is common in both adults and children.

WHO DEVELOPS ALLERGIC RHINITIS?

A high percentage of allergic individuals are children. *Perennial allergic rhinitis* usually manifests before the age of 10 years, while seasonal allergic rhinitis occurs more commonly in teenagers and young adult males. Most patients (10-20% of the population) who present the following symptoms during spring have allergies to seasonal pollens.

SYMPTOMS
• Sneezing
• Congestion
• Runny and itchy nose (rhinitis)
• Postnasal drip
• Itchy red eyes (conjunctivitis)

Development of allergy depends on following:
- Genetics - Is there a family history of allergy?
- Environmental - Is the individual old enough and been exposed to enough pollen?

Symptoms due to allergies may be severe enough to cause loss of time from work and school.

WHAT IS AN ALLERGIC REACTION?

Allergic rhinitis occurs in "atopic" youngsters usually with *normal blood levels of IgE antibodies* to the common inhalant allergens such as house dust mites, tree and grass pollen, animal cockroaches and mould spores. Occasionally food like milk & its products can cause worsening of symptoms. Children are sensitized in early life but may only manifest their allergic symptoms later in life.

The allergic reaction in the nose involves a complex interaction between various inhalant allergens and immune cells. An allergen links with specific IgE antibodies on mast cells near the nasal surface, resulting in release of histamine. This is termed the *immediate allergic reaction*. Other chemicals released by mast cells include thyplase and prostaglandin. Histamine has a direct effect on nasal blood vessels causing swelling and nasal obstruction. It also has a reflex effect via sensory nerves causing sneezing, itching and further mucus production. This triggers a sequence of events with sneezing followed by watery nasal discharge and finally nasal blockage.

Subsequent nasal symptoms that develop between 3 to 12 hours after the initial allergen exposure are termed *late phase reaction*. Further immunity mediator production occurs in the already inflamed nasal membranes and cells (eosinophils and basophils) infiltrate causing progressive nasal blockage and swelling.

Perennial Allergic Rhinitis

Hence, the primary sensitization results in the production of specific IgE antibodies, which later cross-link with allergens on mast cells in the nasal membranes releasing histamine and the allergy cascade. If the condition becomes more entrenched as in *chronic perennial rhinitis*, then other inflammatory mediators and immune cells get involved.

REFERENCES
1. http://www.allergy-clinic.co.uk/hayfever.htm
2. http:/www.allergyhealthcare.com/article%2013.htm

CHAPTER 6

Non-allergic Rhinitis–Types, Description and Clinical Features

Synonyms and Related Keywords

Rhinorrhea, sneezing, pruritus, congestion, infectious rhinitis, non-allergic rhinitis with eosinophil syndrome, (NARES). Occupational rhinitis, hormonal rhinitis, drug-induced rhinitis, gustatory rhinitis and vasomotor rhinitis.

Interestingly, a percentage of patients with classical allergic rhinitis symptoms will be absolutely negative on skin testing. Anti allergic injections are not indicated because these patients are not allergic. And yet patients are just as symptomatic, and just as miserable as the allergic rhinitis patients.

The major manifestations of rhinitis include nasal pruritus, clear rhinorrhea, post-nasal drip and nasal obstruction caused by inflammation of the nasal mucous membranes.

TYPES OF NON-ALLERGIC RHINITIS

1. Vasomotor (the most common form)
2. NARES (Non-allergic Rhinitis with Eosinophilia Syndrome)
3. Drug induced
4. Hormonal
5. Infectious (common cold)

6. Occupational
7. Structural
8. Gustatory

Thus, *in contrast to allergic rhinitis, the common types of non-allergic rhinitis are triggered by irritants and not by allergens.* (In structural rhinitis, the cause is due to structural abnormalities.) *The symptoms of allergic and non-allergic rhinitis overlap significantly, but the cause appears to be entirely different.* Non-allergic rhinitis, a diagnosis of exclusion and it can be sporadic or perennial. It includes a highly diverse group of rhinitis syndromes united by the symptoms of clear rhinorrhea or congestion with less prominent sneezing, nasal pruritus and conjunctival irritation.

Exposure of *non-allergenic irritants* such as dusts, perfume, tobacco smoke, ozone, sulphur dioxide, nitrogen dioxide, cold air and other environmental pollutants produce *nasal hypersensitivity.* This increases the nasal membrane nerve excitability, and results in more mast cells in the superficial nasal membrane. The nasal irritability is so intensified that the patient is affected even by low doses of allergens.

As the lining of the nose and paranasal sinuses are continuous, it is rare for inflammation to affect one without affecting the other. As such, the description *rhinosinusitis* is often mere appropriate.

1. Vasomotor Rhinitis (VMR)–*Most Common* form of Non-Allergic Rhinitis.

"Vaso" means blood vessels and "motor" refers to the nerves, which innervates nasal tissue and the blood vessels. Vasomotor rhinitis (VMR) is a condition is which the tiny blood vessels lining the nose (vaso) may swell and make the nose stuffy, and the mucus glands in the nose may be overactive (motor), leading to excessive running of the nose or post-nasal discharge. The discharge may be thin and watery, and run primarily from the front of the nose or it may be quite thick and chronic, draining down the throat posteriorly, leading to cough, hoarseness, or throat irritation. The phlegm may be quite difficult to clear, particularly upon first waking in the morning.

Vasomotor rhinitis is also referred to as irritant rhinitis. Infections are not involved in vasomotor rhinitis. Usually, however, they are more severe and occur predominantly on one side of the nose. Many cases are associated with a agent or condition. Example of such agents/conditions are:

Potential Triggers of Vasomotor Rhinitis (VMR)
- Changes in temperature or barometric pressure and turbulent air.
- Perfumes; hair spray and cosmetics
- Strong cooking odors and spicy foods
- Cigarette smoke
- Car exhaust and pollution
- Other chemical-based airborne irritants
- Detergents and cleaning solutions
- Chlorine in pools
- Alcoholic beverages
- Inorganic dust (different from dust mite)
- Sexual arousal
- Stress (emotional or physical)

Vasomotor Rhinitis V/S Allergic Rhinitis
- VMR is a *non-specific response* to virtually any change or impurity in the air, as compared to allergic rhinitis (or hay fever), which involves response to a specific protein in pollen, dust, mould or animal dander.

- Symptoms of VMR are similar to those of allergies, with frequent or chronic running of nose, nasal congestion, sneezing episodes and/or post-nasal discharge.
- Patients with VMR, may have less sneezing and itching then the allergic patients.
- In some patients, both conditions may co-exist and the two may aggravate each other. Mixed allergic and non-allergic rhinitis probably account for the majority of cases. This is an important category to recognize, because allergen avoidance measures alone will give only sub-optimal improvements.

SYMPTOMS

- Profuse watery rhinorrhea.
- Nasal obstruction
- Sneezing
- Subjects with vasomotor rhinitis fall into *two general groups:*
    "Runners" who have *"wet"* rhinorrhea, and *"dry"* subjects with predominant symptoms of nasal congestion and blockage to airflow and minimal rhinorrhea.

On Examination
- Congested nasal mucosa
- Snotty nose
- Symptoms disproportional to nasal pathology when examined

Key Features of Vasomotor Rhinitis
- VMR can occur at any age, although it tends to be more common as people get older. It is usually not inherited

- There is usually no history of allergies and irritant may or may not be identified by the patient
- There is no infection causing these symptoms
- Vasomotor rhinitis can have a variable presentation
- Most patients seem to be older than the typical patients with hay fever
- Can sometimes present with a seasonal pattern due to changes in temperature and humidity
- Patients present with rhinorrhea (thick or scanty), frontal headaches and congested turbinates but usually no (itching) pruritus
- Some patients will find that eating especially, spicy foods causes more nasal discharge or congestion.

Other types of non-allergic rhinitis which are less common, are as follows:

2. Non-allergic Rhinitis with Eosinophilia Syndrome (NARES)

A distinguishing feature of NARES is the presence of eosinophils, in nasal smear. It is triggered by environmental changes such as weather or atmospheric changes. The symptoms mimic those of perennial allergic rhinitis. Diagnosis is made after skin tests prove to be negative and a nasal smear reveals the presence of eosinophils. Nasal polyps may also be present.

- Generally, patients with NARES present with nasal congestion, sneezing, rhinorrhea, nasal pruritus and hyposmia.

(According to researchers, elevated eosinophil counts are present in approximately 20% of the general population's nasal smears. However, *not everyone with eosinophilia has symptoms of rhinitis*).

3. Drug-Induced Rhinitis

Drug-induced rhinitis is caused by several medications including decongestant nasal sprays, angiotensin-converting enzyme inhibitors, reserpine, guanethidine, phentolamine, methyldopa, beta-blockers, chlorpromazine, gabapentin, penicillamine, aspirin, non-steroidal anti-inflammatory dugs, inhaled cocaine, exogenous estrogens and oral contraceptives.

Rhinitis medicamentosa is considered a drug-induced rhinitis and results from *prolonged use (i.e. longer than 5-10 days) of topical nasal sympathomimetics.*

Typically, these patients present with extensive nasal congestion and rhinorrhea, resulting from loss of a sympathetic nerve tone, rather than from the original cause of rhinitis. Normal nasal function should resume within 7-21 days following cessation of *sympathomimetics.*

4. Hormonal Rhinitis

Hormonal rhinitis is usually caused by hormonal imbalances as a result of pregnancy, puberty, oral contraceptive conjugated estrogen use and untreated thyroid problem such a hypothyroid states. Estrogen is believed to cause an increase in hyaluronic acid in the nasal mucosa.

- Nasal congestion and rhinorrhea are the chief manifesting symptoms in hormonal rhinitis.
- Initial presentation of *hormonal rhinitis in pregnancy* usually occurs during the second month, continues throughout pregnancy and ceases following delivery.
- Rhinitis associated with pregnancy, is temporary and usually resolves after pregnancy.
- In patients with hypothyroidism, edema increases in the turbinates as a result of thyrotropic hormone release.

- Thyroid replacement therapy will diminish symptoms associated with hypothyroidism.

5. Infectious Rhinitis/Common Cold

Infectious rhinitis occurs due to upper respiratory tract infection *such as common cold*. The nasal discharge is not watery or clear, but thicker with a green tint. Infectious rhinitis is usually caused by an upper respiratory tract infection, either of viral or bacterial origin. Viral infections are generally self-limited and resolve within 7-10 days. However, bacterial infections require the use of antibiotics.

Typically, patients with infectious rhinitis present with *mucopurulent nasal discharge*, rather then watery rhinorrhea, accompanied by facial pain and pressure, altered sense of smell and post-nasal drainage with cough.

6. Occupational Rhinitis

Patients with occupational rhinitis experience symptoms of rhinitis *only at the workplace*. These symptoms are usually initiated as a result of an inhaled irritant (e.g. laboratory animal antigens, grains, wood dusts and chemicals). Frequently, patiently with occupational rhinitis present with occupational asthma.

7. Structural Rhinitis

Structural rhinitis is caused by structural abnormalities such as a *deviated nasal septum or a broken nose*. This type of rhinitis usually affects one side of the nose more than the other. Surgery may be needed to correct the abnormality and for relief of symbloms.

8. Gustatory Rhinitis

This type of rhinitis occurs following consumption of hot and spicy foods. This present with a "wet" (profuse watery) nose, secondary to nasal vasodilatation (dilated blood vessels) and is due to stimulation of the vagus nerve, generally occurring within a few hours of eating the food.

REFERENCES

1. http://www.allergyclinic.co.nz/guides/50.html
2. http://www.emedicine.com/ent/topic402.htm
3. http://www.regionalallergy.com/vmrinfo.htm
4. http://www.astelin.com./rhinitisproblem/screener.html
5. http://www.allergylealthcare.com/article%2013.thm

CHAPTER 7

Etiology of Chronic Non-allergic Idiopathic Rhinitis

A wide variety causations are involved in non-allergic rhinitis. Therefore, treatment options should not be implemented randomly and should be aimed *primarily at resolving underlying causative factors*. Rhinitis is inflammation of the lining of the nose, which may be caused by allergies of other factors. But nasal inflammation is not always-related. There are many forms of rhinitis that do not have IgE responses.

Rhinitis can be either acute or chronic. Non-allergic rhinitis occurs in those patients in whom allergic causes cannot be identified. Some types of non-allergic rhinitis are triggered by a number of irritants, but these are not allergens and there is no evidence of an allergic response. For instance, vasomotor rhinitis is thought to occur because of abnormal regulation of nasal blood flow. Mixed allergic and non-allergic, rhinitis, probably, account for the majority of cases. This is an important category to recognize, as allergen avoidance measures alone will give unsatisfactory results.

CAUSATIVE FACTORS FOR NON-ALLERGIC RHINITIS

1. Non- Allergic Immune Response (e.g. NARES)

Some cases of chronic rhinitis are associated with *increase in number* of *eosinophils*. These are components of the immune system that releases powerful inflammatory factors and produce nasal congestion in susceptible people. These immune factors are not related to the allergic response, although they can be triggered by several factors including environmental changes such as weather or atmospheric changes, cigarette smoke, other air pollutants, strong odors, alcoholic beverages, and exposure to cold. An example of this type of rhinitis is *Non-allergic rhinitis with eosinophilia syndrome (NARES)*.

2. Irritants

Congestion and stuffy nose may occur in response to irritants, including smoke, environmental toxins, changes in temperature and humidity, stress, and even sexual. Such triggers are numerous:

- Air Pollution; cigarette smoke and car exhaust fumes.
- Alcoholic beverages and spicy foods.
- Chemicals; cleaning solutions and laundry detergents.
- Emotional upsets
- Perfumes; strong odors and cosmetics

This over-reaction causes swelling in the nasal passages but is not associated with any immune response. This is known as *vasomotor rhinitis,* also referred to as irritant rhinitis. The biological causes are unknown. According to a research, an *association exists between vasomotor rhinitis and gastro-esophageal reflux disorder (GERD,* a common cause of heartburn), which some experts feel may be, due to a *common defect in the nervous system that controls muscle action.*

3. Aging Process in the Elderly

The elderly are at risk for chronic rhinitis as the mucous membranes become dry with age. In addition, the cartilage supporting the nasal passages weakens, causing changes in airflow.

In such cases, therapy involves avoiding possible allergens and airborne irritants as well as measures to keep the nasal passages moist. (Decongestants would not be appropriate). Another cause is sensitivity to temperature changes.

"Old man's drip"- hyper-reactivity to small changes in temperature in elderly men (may respond to testosterone).

4. Structural Abnormalities

A number of conditions may block the nasal passages resulting in *structural rhinitis*. Surgery may be helpful for certain cases to correct the abnormality.

Deviated Septum

A common structural abnormality that causes rhinitis is a deviated septum. The septum is the inner wall of cartilage and bone that separates the two sides of the nose. When it is deviated, it is not straight but shifted to one side, usually the left. A deviation in the septum of the nose can cause narrowing of the nasal passage resulting in congestion.

Other Causes of Blockage

Rarely, cleft palates, broken nose, overgrowth of bones in the nose, or tumors cause rhinitis.

5. Medications and illegal Drugs

A number of drugs can cause rhinitis or worsen it in people with pre-existing conditions such as deviated septum, allergies or vasomotor rhinitis. These are listed below:

Decongestants

Overuse of decongestant sprays used to treat nasal congestion can, over time (three to five days), cause inflammation in the nasal passages and worsen rhinitis.

NSAIDS

Many people with allergies and asthma are sensitive to some of the common pain killers known as *non-steroidal anti-inflammatory drugs* (NSAIDS). They include the common drugs aspirin, ibuprofen (Motrin, Advil, Nuprin, Rufen), and naproxen (Aleve) among many others. Aspirin and products containing aspirin, can even cause life threatening asthma attacks in some highly susceptible individuals.

Adrenergic Neurone Blocking Agents

e.g. guanethidine.

Other Medications

That may cause rhinitis include oral contraceptives, hormone replacement therapy, anti-anxiety agents (particularly alprazolam), some antidepressants, and some blood pressure medications, including beta-blockers.

Peripheral Vasodilators

As used in the treatment of migraine and peripheral vascular disease.

Cocaine

Sniffing cocaine damages nasal passages and can cause chronic rhinitis.

6. Estrogen in Women

- *Elevated levels of estrogen appear to increase mucus production and swelling in the nasal passages and can cause congestion.* This effect is most apparent in women during pregnancy. In such cases the condition usually clears up after delivery.
- Oral contraceptives and hormone replacement therapies that contain estrogen have also been associated with nasal congestion in some women.

Etiology of Chronic Non-allergic Idiopathic Rhinitis

7. Susceptibility to Infections (Non-Allergic Rhinitis in Children)

Chronic nasal congestion in children often accompanies a susceptibility to ear, sinus, or adenoid infections. Adenoids are spongy tissue masses located between ends of the nasal passages and the soft tissue in the back of the throat. Enlarged adenoids may also cause ear problems. The bacteria that cause these infections, however, are not usually the cause of this chronic rhinitis.

8. Foreign Objects

Blockage in young children is often caused by foreign objects that they have pushed up in their nose. If they are left in place, they may eventually cause infection and nasal discharge, usually in one side of the nose, which may be yellow or green with foul smell.

9. Nasal Polyps

In some people, nasal polyps can cause congestion and sometimes, loss of sense of smell. These are soft, gray, fluid-filled sacs that develop stalk-like structures on the mucus membrane. They impede mucus drainage and restrict airflow. Polyps develop from sinus infections that cause overgrowth of the mucus membrane in the nose. They do not regress on their own and in fact, may multiply and cause considerable obstruction. Nasal polyps are associated with aspirin sensitivity. They can be surgically removed but often grow back.

10. Other Medical Conditions

- *Hypothyroidism* is associated with chronic rhinitis.
- People with certain genetic or other medical conditions that specifically affect the mucous membranes are also at risk, although rhinitis in such people is apt to be only

one of the many more serious conditions, including chronic sinusitis and respiratory problems.

- *Wegener's granulomatosis*, for example, is a serious but very rare illness that causes long-term swelling and tumor-like masses in air passages.
- *Rare genetic disorders* that cause chronic rhinitis include the following:

    Cystic fibrosis, in which the mucus is very thick.

    Kartagener's syndrome in which the body's major internal organs are located in the mirror-image position of their normal location. In addition, the body's cilia (hair-like/projections on many body tissues that help to move mucus and other fluids) are motionless. In both disorders, mucus build-up therefore produces an environment favourable for infection caused by organisms.

11. Emotional Factors

Autonomic imbalance due to emotions such as stress and sexual arousal.

REFERENCES
1. http://www.umm.edu/patiented/what_rhinitis_000077 _1.
2. httm://allergic.about.com/cs/other/a/aa052002a.htm
3. http://www.emedicine.com/ent/topic402/htm
4. httm://www.gpnotebook.co.uk/simplepage.cfm?iD=-972685262&linkID=29895&cook=yes

CHAPTER 8

Pathophysiology of Non Allergic/ Idiopathic Rhinitis

Rhinitis is basically an inflammation of the inner lining of the nose. *Pathophysiology* of allergic rhinitis is easier to understand since the role of allergens is well defined, in contrast to non-allergic rhinitis where no cause can be identified. For instance, vasomotor rhinitis (a common type of non-allergic rhinitis) is thought to occur because of abnormal regulation of nasal blood flow. There appears to be an imbalance in the function of nerves that make mucous glands secrete fluid and which causes blood vessels to swell or contract.

WHAT HAPPENS IN ALLERGIC RHINITIS?

The allergic reaction in the nose involves a complex interaction between various inhalant allergens and immune cells. An allergen will link to specific *IgE antibodies* on mast cells near the nasal surface resulting in histamine release. This is termed the; immediate allergic reaction. Other chemicals released by mast cells include tryptase and prostaglandin. Histamine has a direct effect on nasal blood vessels causing swelling and nasal obstruction. It also has a reflex effect via sensory nerves causing sneezing, itching and further mucus production. This triggers a sequence of events with sneezing followed by watery nasal discharge and finally nasal blockage. Subsequent nasal symptoms that develop between 3 and 12 hours after the initial allergen exposure are due to the 'late phase reaction'.

DIFFERENT TYPES OF NON-ALLERGIC RHINITIS

Non-allergic rhinitis affects 5-10% of the population. However, only 2-4% of patients actually seek treatment for relief of their symptoms. Patients may or may not present with the same symptomses seen in allergic rhinitis.

As seen earlier, *non-allergic rhinitis has 7 basic sub-classifications,* including:

Infectious rhinitis (common cold)

Non-allergic rhinitis with eosinophilia syndromes (NARES)

Occupational rhinitis

Hormonal rhinitis

Drug-induced rhinitis

Gustatory rhinitis

Vasomotor rhinitis

Among these, *the most common form of non-allergic rhinitis is the vasomotor rhinitis* which is an *incompletely understood disorder* that involves a disturbance in the way the parasympathetic nervous system and controls the blood vessels in the nose.

DEFINITION AND PATHOPHYSIOLOGY OF NON-ALLERGIC RHINITIS

Non-allergic rhinitis is characterized by sporadic or persistent perennial symptoms of rhinitis that do not result from IgE-mediated immunopathologic events. The diagnosis of rhinitis without positive skin tests falls under two common subgroups:

One subgroup, non-allergic rhinitis with eosinophilia syndrome (NARES), presents with allergic symptoms in addition to conditions such as nasal polyps and nasal eosinophilia (cells called eosinophils are present in nasal mucosa), asthma and frequently sinusitis.

The other subgroup, vasomotor rhinitis, presents with symptoms, especially congestion, but other associated conditions may not be so intense.

The nasal mucosal lining has a rich blood supply that is control of the autonomic nervous system. Non-specific stimuli may act on the autonomic nervous system. Such non-specific stimuli include rapid changes in weather, temperature and humidity, drafts, exposure to chemicals, odors, perfumes, smoke and dust, emotions or stress, which may increase blood flow to the tissue resulting in swelling, congestion and rhinitis.

Less Common Subgroups

There are also patients who come under other less common subgroups. A significantly *deviated septum* may also induce changes in the mucosa, worsen the non-allergic or vasomotor rhinitis and increase nasal congestion and drainage. Although the exact mechanism is unknown, hormonal changes that occur with pregnancy, menstruation, menopause, hypothyroidism and oral contraceptives may cause symptoms of chronic non-allergic rhinitis.

Patients complain of chronic nasal congestion, rhinitis, postnasal drip and sneezing. *Congestion and blockage may alternate from side to side* and are usually constant, though *seasonal weather changes (during the spring and may trigger symptoms that mimic pollen or dust allergies*. Symptoms may worsen upon awakening in the morning. Examination reveals marked pink or pale nasal swelling, obstruction and thick nasal secretion. In all cases, *skin tests are negative*. Patients with non-allergic but not vasomotor rhinitis will have eosinophils present in nasal secretions and frequently, nasal polyps complicating the obstruction.

ABSENCE OF IMMUNOGLOBULIN E (IOE)

Non-allergic rhinitis is basically a diagnosis of rhinitis without any immunoglobulin (IgE) mediation as documented by allergen skin testing. Hence, rhinorrhea, sneezing, pruritus, and congestion do not result from allergy or hypersensitivity and continue to persist, whether continuously or sporadically.

IMMUNOGLOBULIN G (IOG)

Elevated concentrations of immunoglobulin G sub-class 1 (IgG1), immunoglobulin G sub-class 4 (IgG4) and anti-IgE autoantibodies have been found in patients with non-allergic rhinitis relative to concentrations found in placebo patients. *However, these elevations are lower than those found in patients with allergic rhinitis.* In addition to skin testing, serum-soluble 'Fas' concentrations (inherent signals for causing cell death) are not elevated in patients with non-allergic rhinitis, unlike in patients with allergic rhinitis. Increased concentration of serum-soluble 'Fas' is often present in patients with autoimmune diseases and cancer.

ROLE OF AUTONOMIC NERVOUS SYSTEM IN RHINITIS

The autonomic nervous system controls the blood supply to the nasal mucosa and the secretion of mucus. The diameter of the resistance vessels in the nose is mediated by the sympathetic nervous system while the parasympathetic nervous system controls glandular secretion and to a lesser extent, exerts an effect on the vessels. A *hypoactive sympathetic nervous system* or a *hyperactive parasympathetic nervous system* can engorge these vessels, thereby increasing the swelling of the nasal mucosa, and thus congestion. Activation of the parasympathetic nervous system can also increase mucosal secretions leading to an excess in the running nose.

Evaluation of the Autonomic Nervous system Patients with Vasomotor Rhinitis (VMR)

Vasomotor rhinitis is the most common type of non-allergic rhinitis. It has been suspected that vasomotor rhinitis is either due to a hyperactive parasympathetic nervous system or an imbalance between it and the sympathetic nervous system. The exact relation has not been determined. Recently neurological laboratories have been developed in which a series of tests can be performed to determine reactivity of the autonomic nervous system. It is found that *autonomic nervous system dysfunction is significant in patients with vasomotor rhinitis*. Possible factors that trigger this dysfunction may include nasal trauma and extra-esophageal manifestations of gastro-esophageal reflux.

Researchers from the University of Chicago in illinois have reviewed some current concepts in the *pathophysiology* of vasomotor rhinitis. There is emerging evidence that neuropeptides and nitric oxide may play pathogenic roles in VMR. There is also evidence of hypoactive *autonomic sympathetic function* in VMR. Irritants such as ozone and cigarette smoke may trigger neurogenic mechanisms in VMR.

Autonomic Stimuli

Autonomic stimuli have a greater effect on patients with non-allergic rhinitis than on those with allergic rhinitis. Patients can reduce nasal airway resistance up to 50% through isotonic exercise, which is mediated by increases in sympathetic tone. Changes in body posture, from erect to supine position, can also increase nasal airway resistance. In the supine position, the right nostril will have lower pressure relative to the left nostril if the patient lies on the right side. *Temperature can also impact nasal blood flow and compliance. Nasal compliance is decreased with cold air and increased with hot air,* whereas nasal blood flow is independent of changes in hot air but decreases in the presence of cold air.

It is thus clearly evident that non-allergic rhinitis is characterized by sporadic or persistent perennial symptoms of rhinitis that do not result from IgE-mediated immunopathologic events.

CHAPTER 9

Mechanisms Operating in Different Forms of Non-allergic Rhinitis

It may be pointed out that the mechanism in each type of rhinitis is rather poorly understood. Non-allergic rhinitis may occur with or without other complications.

1. NARES (Non-allergic Rhinitis with Eosinophilia Syndrome)

Non-allergic rhinitis with eosinophilia syndrome (NARES) is characterized by nasal congestion and *prominent nasal eosinophilia*. The mechanism of the eosinophil infiltration is not known. Eosinophilia is also prominent in following conditions:
- When nasal polyps are present, but again the mechanism of eosinophil recruitment is not know.
- In patients with aspirin sensitivity.

2. Hormonal Rhinitis

There are several causes of non-allergic rhinitis without inflammation/inflammatory cells. *Endocrine changes of hypothyroid and hyperthyroid disease*, and pregnancy can lead to unremitting nasal congestion.
- Damage to sympathetic nerves, as in Horner's syndrome, can oblate sympathetic vasoconstrictor tone and lead to unopposed vasodilatory parasympathetic reflexes and chronic nasal congestion.

- In patients with hypothyroidism edema increases in the 'turbinates' as a result of thyrotropic hormone release.

3. Vasomotor Rhinitis

Vasomotor rhinitis is the inflamation of the nose nosal mucosa due to *abnormal neuronal control* of the blood vessels the nose. It is a non-specific response to virtually any change or impurity in the air, as opposed to allergic rhinitis (or hay fever), which involves a response to a *specific protein* in pollen, dust, mould or animal dander. Any strong odor or any particulate matter in the air, including pollens, dust, mould, or animal dander can bother people with VMR, even though they are not actually allergic to these things.

As described above earlier subjects with vasomotor rhinitis fall into two general groups: "*runners*" who have "*wet*" rhinorrhea, and "*dry*" subjects with predominant symptoms of nasal congestion and blockage to airflow, and minimal rhinorrhea. These reactions can be provoked by non-specific irritant stimuli such as cold dry air, perfumes, paint, fumes and cigarette smoke indicating that over-active irritant receptors may also play a role in vasomotor rhinitis.

Subjects with surface predominantly from rhinorrhea (sometimes referred to as cholinergic rhinitis) appear to have enhanced cholinergic glandular secretory activity, since atropine effectively reduces their secretions. Subjects with predominan nasal congestion and blockage may have nociceptive neurons that have heightened sensitivity to innocuous stimuli.

4. Drug-induced Rhinitis

Overuse of topical nasal decongestants also leads to chronic nasal congestion ("rhinitis medicamentosa"). During this process, the alpha-receptors in the nose are gradually desensitized to endogenous and exogenous stimulation. Typically, these patient presents with extensive nasal congestion and rhinorrhea, resulting from loss of adrenergic tone, rather than from the original cause of rhinitis.

5. Gustatory Rhinitis

Some patients find that eating causes more nasal drainage or congestion. This is because the digestive process includes the production of mucus in the gastrointestinal tract. The nerves and reflexes that control this are very closely related to the nerves that control the nose, and sometimes this reaction of mucus production "*spills over*" to the nose when eating. This is normal with all people, to a certain extent, with spicy and cold/frozen foods.

CHAPTER 10

Complications of Persistent or Recurring Rhinitis

IMPAIRED QUALITY OF LIFE

The chief long-term disadvantage is the impaired quality of life resulting in frustration since the patient is unable to carry on with his/her daily activities. *Congestion, sneezing and constant nose blowing* can cause discomfort and social embarrassment. The resulting *sleeplessness, fatigue and irritability* can also affect the patient's performance at work or school.

Persistent rhinitis can lead to related disorders such as:

Learning Impairment in Children

Children with rhinitis may suffer learning impairment due to annoying symptoms, and daytime fatigue from sleep loss.

Chronic Sinusitis

A common complication, which occurs in individuals with rhinitis is infection of sinuses. Since the sinus openings may be blocked due to chronic swelling, the sinuses will not drain properly. The mucus drip may plug the sinus passages, leading to sinus infection and pain.

- *This infection can present as toothache facial fullness or discharge.* Prolonged sinus congestion also causes pain, tenderness and swelling around eyes, cheeks, nose or forehead and can be either acute or chronic.

Hearing Loss

Dysfunction of the eustachian tubes that connect the ear to the throat resulting in temporary hearing loss.

Otitis Media (Middle Ear Infection)

The mucus drainage may plug the tube between the nose and the ear, causing an ear infection and pain. Rhinitis is often a contributing factor for middle ear infection (otitis media), which causes pain, fever and fluid buid up in the middle ear. Children are especially vulnerable to this infection.

Aggravation of Asthma

Rhinitis may increase the risk of developing or aggravating serious asthma.

Structural Changes

Structural deformities like high arched palate.

Nasal Drainage

Drainage from inflamed or infected sinuses may be thick or discolored.

Post-nasal Drip

Excessive mucus production may run down the back of the throat or cause a cough that is usually worse at night.

Persistent Sore Throat

May also result from excessive mucus drainage.

REFERENCES

1. http://www.aaaai.org/aadmc/currentliterature/selectedarticles/2004archive/vasomctor_rhinitis
2. http://www.allergy clinic.co.uk/hayfever.htm
3. http://www.icaai.org/Param/Rhinitis/Complete/non_allergic_thi iitis.htm
4. http://www.regonalallergy.com/vmrinfo.htm

CHAPTER **11**

Non-allergic Rhinitis in Special Cases

A cautious approach is highly recommended while treating special cases such as:
- Children
- Elderly patients
- Pregnant or nursing women
- Athletes
- Patients with renal / hepatic insufficiency

Oral anti-histamines, nasal sprays and other medications are known to have side effects and it is wiser to avoid or minimize their use. The undesirable side effects like sedation and fatigue associated with some oral antihistamines are well known.

I. CHILDREN

Non-allergic rhinitis (of all types) is not very common in children. Even children presenting with NARES account for less than 2% of children with nasal eosinophilia. It is recommended that preventive and non-pharmacologic approaches should be tried before beginning medication in children.

If possible, first-generation oral antihistamines should be avoided to prevent adverse reaction, particularly paroxysmal hyperactivity.

Nasal corticosteroids are sometimes used for pediatric

patients presenting with rhinorrhea, sneezing, pruritus and congestion. FDA recommends routine monitoring of height in children treated with corticosteroids.

Certain corticosteroids such as *beclomethasone* (Beclovent), are not recommended for children younger than six years because continued growth suppression. In adults, traditional oral antihistamines and newer less-sedating anti-histamines have no established beneficial effects on decongestants can cause irritation and 'rhinitis medicamentosa' without proven benefit.

II. PREGNANT WOMEN

Symptoms of rhinitis can increase during pregnancy. This increase is thought to be caused by progesterone and estrogen induced glandular secretion, augmented by nasal vascular pooling from vasodilation and increased blood volume. The rhinitis associated with pregnancy is temporary and usually resolves after pregnancy.

In pregnant females who present with symptoms of rhinitis the diagnosis should not be limited to hormonal rhinitis. *The cause can be 'rhinitis medicamentosa',* an if so, patient needs to be weaned from topical sympathomimetics. Pregnancy may also be complicated by infectious rhinitis, which may require the use of antibiotics. Additionally, some patients may present with vasomotor rhinitis. Nasal saline solution and exercise are usually beneficial in these cases. Vasomotor rhinitis in pregnancy respond well to intranasal saline instillation.

Caution in Using Some Common Medications During Pregnancy and Lactation

It is advisable to avoid or minimize the use of medications such as antihistamines, nasal steroidal sprays and sympathomimetics, during pregnancy and lactation. If at all necessary, they have to be used with extreme caution. Potential risks versus benefits should be considered in the use of FDA-approved topical anticholinergics (pregnancy category B), topical anti-histamines (pregnancy category C), and topical corticosteroids (pregnancy category C). No conclusive data has been published for use of any inhaled corticosteroids during lactation and breast-feeding.

Patients should exercise caution if taking antihistamines while breast-feeding. These drugs are also likely to reduce the milk volume in lactating women. Both topical and systemic sympathomimetics are rated as pregnancy category C. These drugs act as powerful vasoconstrictors therefore potential exists for uterine blood flow reduction. These drugs are also excreted in breast milk,

III. ATHLETES

Althletes with non-allergic rhinitis who actively compete on state and national levels may be difficult to treat. Athletes are not permitted to use any oral decongestants. Each sporting event is likely to have its own regulations. The prescribing physician should verify accepted medications in advance through written communication to the appropriate supervising committees. The stepwise approach to manage athletes should be the same as that used with other populations.

IV. ELDERLY PATIENTS

Cholinergic and alpha-adrenergic hyperactivity are common causes of rhinitis in elderly patients. The increased cholinergic respones in part may be the result of activation by various foods (i.e. gustatory rhinitis). While nasal sprays may seem to be the obvious choice for this type of watery rhinorrhea, some elderly patients may be troubled by unwanted side effects, particularly loss of bladder control.

Three types of non-allergic rhinitis commonly occur in older patients.

- The first type vasomotor rhinitis, is thought to be caused by increased cholinergic activity and is similar to that occurring in younger patients. Symptoms of vasomotor rhinitis may be exacerbated by certain odors, alcohol, spicy foods, emotions and environmental factors.
- The second type, gustatory rhinitis, is associated with profuse, watery rhinorrhea that may be exacerbated by eating.
- The third type is believed to arise from alpha-adrenergic hyperactivity, stimulated by the regular use of anti-hypertensives.

V. RENAL/HEPATIC INSUFFICIENCY

Patients with renal insufficiency, hepatic insufficiency or both are prone to augmentation of adverse events, resulting from a reduced clearance through these pathways. Intranasal admininistration is considered safer.

REFERENCES

1. http://www.emedicine.com/ent/topic402/htm
2. http://www.aafp.org/afp/20050915/1057.html

CHAPTER 12

Diagnostic Tests

Diagnostic tests which are given below may sometimes be required while dealing with persistent or recurring cases of rhinitis. Diagnosis is also useful in terms of *case management and prognosis.*

1. Physical Examination

The inside of the nose can be examined with a torch and speculum. This is painless examination and allows the doctor to check for *signs of inflammation.* The eyes, ears, and chest should be examined too.

Simple rhinoscopy or nasal examination using a good light-source may also reveal; pale bluish swollen nasal membranes, moist discharge and occasional evidence of *polyps.*

2. Skin Tests for Allergy

A skin test is a simple method for detecting common allergens. Patients are usually tested for a panel of common allergens. Skin tests are rarely needed to diagnose mild seasonal allergic rhinitis, since the cause is usually obvious. The test is not appropriate for children under three years of age.

The procedure is as follows:

- Patients should not take anti-histamines for at least 12 to 72 hours before the test. Otherwise an allergic reaction may not show up.

- Small amounts of suspected allergens are applied to the skin with a needle prick or scratch (,i.e. *epicutaneous test*).
- Small amounts of suspected allergens are injected a few cells deep into the skin (,i.e. *intradermal test*). This test is more sensitive than the standard prick test.
- If an allergy in present, a hive (a swollen reddened area) is formed within about 20 minutes.
- Occasionally, skin prick test reactions are found mildly positive in patients with VMR, but it does not fit the history and is therefore not relevant to the cause of rhinitis.

The skin test is *not completely accurate*. For instance, a study conducted in year 2001 reported that tests detected allergies in less than half of children with rhinitis. Furthermore, about 15% to 20% of people may have a skin reaction without actually having an allergy.

3. Laboratory Tests

Nasal Smear

The physician may take a nasal smear. The nasal secretion is examined microscopically for factors that might indicate a cause, such as in increased number of white blood cells, indicating infection, or high counts of eosinophils. (*High eosinophil counts indicate an allergic condition,* but low count does not rule out allergic rhinitis).

Blood Test

Blood tests can also detect allergens, but blood tests are generally less sensitive than skin tests. Allergic rhinitis is diagnosed when specific antigens can be identified and is often sub-classified as seasonal or perennial allergic rhinitis.

Eosinophil detection

A useful laboratory test in rhinitis is to take a nasal mucus sample and test for eosinophils using Hansel's Stain. If *plenty of eosinophil cells* are present, this provides indication towards the diagnosis of allergic rhinitis.

Tests for IgE

Tests for IgE immunoglobulin production in blood may also be performed. One is called the Radio-allergo-sorbent Test (RAST) is used to detect increased levels of *allergen-specific IgE* in response to particular allergens. Bloood tests for IgE may be less accurate than skin tests. They should only be performed on patients who cannot undergo skin testing or when skin test results are uncertain.

4. Imaging Tests

In people with chronic rhinitis, the physician may also check for sinusitis. Imaging tests may be useful if other tests are ambiguous.

- A test called transillumination, this physician shines a bright light against the patient's cheek or forehead. (is an enexpensive method for checking abnormalities in the sinus cavities, although not highly accurate).
- X-rays of the skull and sinuses.
- CT scans of the head: In some cases, a CT scan of the sinuses may be required to exclude chronic sinusitis or polyposis. **Radiology** (X-rays sinus and CAT scan) does not help in the diagnosis of allergic rhinitis, but will identify complications such as chronic sinusitis, infections, nasal polyps and sinus fluid levels.

5. Nasal Endoscopy

In certain cases of chronic or unresponsive rhinitis, a physician may use endoscope to examine for any irregularities in the nose structure. Endoscope which contains instruments and a miniature camera is inserted to view the passeges.

6. Other Diagnostic Tests

- **Nitric oxide (NO)** – The levels of NO in expired air tends to be higher in patients suffering with allergic inflammation of nasal mclosa. This test in useful to detect degree of inflammation in cases of chronic rhinitis.
- **Fibre-optic Nasal Endoscopes** - ENT specialist and surgeons make use of fibre-optic nasal endoscopes to visualise the nasal membran septum and osteo-meatal complex of the nasal sinuses.
- **Rhino-manometry** - It is a measure of nasal air flow, *nasal provocation tests* with the chemical histamine and microscopy of nasal mucus specimens are more useful for research purposes.

In practice, allergic rhinitis is excluded or implicated as the cause of symptoms by using conventional skin testing or by evaluation for specific IgE antibodies to know allergens.

CHAPTER **13**

Differential Diagnosis

Asthma and Sinusitis

Asthma and sinusitis may be associated with rhinitis. It is useful to establish a more specific diagnosis through diagnostic testing since this would help in the management of the case.

Sinusitis

Sinus Infection - May be the cause of the stuffy or the runny nose. The discharge may be thick and possibly discolored. However, it may also be thin and clear. Facial pain tenderness, headache and internal coughing usually accompany a sinus infection. Fever may or may not be present. Halitosis (bad breath) may also indicate sinusitis. Cold or flu symptoms, allergies, or a deviated nasal septum precede sinus infections. An antibiotic may be needed for treatment.

Allergic and Vasomotor Rhinitis

People with allergic rhinitis usually have a positive family history for allergies and usually respond favorably to antihistamines and anti-inflammatory drugs. The individual with vasomotor rhinitis usually does not.

In addition to the historical data to help distinguish allergic from vasomotor rhinitis, allergy testing can be done to differentiate these 2 types of chronic rhinitis. If allergies are ruled out, then vasomotor rhinitis is likely, but, these conditions can co-exist and synergistically increase individual's symptoms.

Infectious Rhinitis

Common Cold or Upper Respiratory Tract Infection - It can be confused with allergic rhinitis, but the presence of eye irritation and the fever generally point to allergic rhinitis. A stuffy or a runny nose is most often a symptom of common cold. The discharge is usually *thin and clear* (it might be a little bloody). With cold, the stuffy or the runny nose is generally accompanied by sneezing, a scratchy feeling in throat and and mild fatigue.

NARES

Profuse symptoms with negative allergy tests, but with the *presence of eosinophil cells in the nasal mucus*. This condition is termed non-allergic rhinitis with eosinophilia syndrome (NARES).

Food Related Rhinitis

Symptoms may be seen in 70% of the infants and young children, but are frequently associated with symptoms of skin or gastrointestinal irritation

Foreign Objects

Foreign objects in the nose (,e.g. peas and bugs) will cause the nose to become stuffy or runny and may lead to rhinitis symptoms. The discharge will range from thick to thin and would be accompanied by a foul/disagreeable smell in the nose and halitosis (bad breath). The foreign object must be removed and may require professional help. Foreign objects in the nose are common only in children and people with significant mental or behavioral disorders.

Vasomotor Rhinitis

This is triggered by *irritants* (,e.g. smoke, smog or dust) or weather changes, often seasonal in nature, but *is not due to an allergy*. The nasal discharge will generally be *clear and thin*.

Anatomical Abnormalities

Such as deviated septum; this is evident on physical examination.

Allergic Rhinitis

A stuffy or a runny nose may be a symptom of allergic rhinitis (allergies). Allergies, such as hay fever, grass fever or rose fever, are the responses of the nose to pollen, moud or house dust. With allergy, there is generally very thin and clear, itching and running for the eyes is usually associated with the allergy induced in nose. Allergic symptoms tend to be either *seasonal* — usually spring fall, year round usually associated with dust allergy, or *sporadic* in response to a specific and relatively rare exposure to an offending substance.

REFERENCES
1. http://www.emedicine.com/ent/topic402.htm
2. http://www.realage.com/home_care/suffy_nose_generated/topic/contect.asp?
3. http://www.umm.edu/patiented/articles/
4. http://www.mayoclinic.com/health/hay-fever/DS00174/DSECTION=6

CHAPTER 14

Life Style and Management Advice to Rhinitis Patients

Life Style Advice

It is often harder to treat non-allergic than rhinitis. This is because there are fewer options; there are no allergens to avoid and immunotherapy injections don't help. It is not always possible to avoid *irritants or allergens*, but exposure to them can be *minimized* in order to keep the symptoms under control.

- Minimize exposure to know *environmental irrtants* such as car exhaust, smoke, etc. Patient should avoid going to areas where the air has a high concentration of such particles. Any type of irritant that is inhaled into the nose may aggravate symptoms.
- During periods of heavy pollution, drive your car with the windows and vent closed.
- Avoid cigarette smoke. It is important that *patients with* vasomotor rhinitis or indeed any respiratory problem should *not smoke actively passively.* Cigarette smoke contains numerous toxic and irrtating particles and gases that aggravate with lining of the nose, increasing both congestion and mucus production. The fine cigarette particles harmful to the respiratory tract stay in air for up to 24 hours and rapidly spread throughout the house.

Therefore, cigarette smoking must not be trochoid in vicinity of patient.

- It is not adequate for other family members to smoke only in a designated room, or to smoke only when the patient is away from home. Even the most sophisticated and powerful air cleaning devices are quickly outpaced by smoke, and are not a substitute for always keeping outdoors.
- Avoid using aerosol products: The thing that aggravate vasomotor rhinitis most specifically is aerosol products. These may include hair sprays, deodorants, insecticides and many others. Use a roll-on deodorant instead of sprays. If hair spray is required, use the pump type.
- If the house has to be treated with insecticide, shift temprarily elsewhere during the applications.
- Close doors and windows during pollen season; stay indoors on sunny and windy days.
- *Use a dehumidifier* to reduce indoor humidity to less then 50 percent.
- If possible, use air conditioning in side the house and car.
- Use a high-efficiency particulate air (HEPA) filler in the bedroom.
- Avoid moving the lawn or raking the leaves, which stris up pollen and moulds.
- Reduce exposure to dust and dust mites by keeping the house clean.
- Minimize exposure to pet dander by keeping pets clean or by avoiding pets.

MANAGEMENT ADVICE - SPECIFIC MEASURES

Chronic non-allergic rhinitis, especially vasomotor rhinitis

Life Style and Management Advice to Rhinitis Patients

can cause much frustration and discomfort. While there is no cure, as of now, for this condition, there are ways to help. As with most chronic problems, the key to control is understanding on the part of the patient.

- Keep the mucus thin rather than, thick and sticky. This helps complications, such as ear and sinus infections, and plugging of your nasal passages.

  To make the mucus thin:
  - Use *saline nasal sprays*
  - Drink extra fluids
  - Increase the humidity in the air with a vaporizer or humidifier

- *Salt water nose spray* may be very useful in vasomotor rhinitis. Use steam or salt water sprays to soothe and unblock the nose.
- Frequent *steam inhalations* can reduce nasal congestion.
- *Restricted diets*: Some people find that certain foods make their nose water or cause sneezing, and may prefer to avoid them.
- *If acid-reflux is also present,* avoid alcohol, caffeine, and late evening meals and snacks. Elevating the head in bed may help to decrease reflux during sleep.
- Some patients derive significant help from either a room or central humidifier, especially in winters when heaters are turned on and the air is very dry.
- Anti-histamines may sometimes be needed to reduce the amount of mucus. But it is necessary to use with caution because some them may cause drowsiness.
- *Avoid chronic use of nasal drops or sprays* (Afrin, Neosynephrine, etc.). It is advisable not to use over-the-

counter nasal sprays more frequently than 3 days. Used consistently, these preparations cause "*rebound swelling*", that is, the more they are used, the more they are needed until they do more harm than good. Hence, it is better not to use these preperations for more than 2-3 days in a row. They may be used as a resort only when really necessary.

- If nasal blockage is a predominant symptom, surgical procedures may alleviate the problem by correcting anatomical abnormalities.

REFERENCES
1. http://www/nlm.nih.gov/medlineplus/ency/article/0013051.htm
2. http://www.emedicine.com/ent/topic402.htm
3. http:www.regionalallergy.com/vmrinfo.htm
4. http://www.mayoclinic.com/health/hay-fever/DS00174/DSECTION=7
5. http://www.otherhealth.com/archive/index.php/t-916/html
6. http://www.allergycapital.com.au/Pages/nar.html

CHAPTER **15**

Conventional Treatment of Non-Allergic Rhinitis and Its Drawbacks

TREATMENT OF NON-ALLERGIC RHINITIS BY CONVENTIONAL MEDICINE

Non-allergic rhinitis is difficut to treat than allergic rhinitis. There is no actual "cure" for non-*allergic rhinitis*. Several medications that are available only help to alleviate symptoms. Unlike allergic rhinitis, there is no specific or preventive therapy, such as anti-allergy injection, to permanently reduce the body's sensitivity to triggering factors. Avoidance of the irritant is the most successful treatment. But it is also harder to avoid the triggers of recurring rhinitis like vasomotor rhinitis.

Treatment of chronic rhinitis and post-nasal drip depends on the underlying condition causing the problem. A complete history and examination is done to determine if the problem is caused by either an impairment in the normal production of mucus or in its normal clearance from the nose.

TREATMENT

Consist of one of more of the following.
- Avoiding environmental irritants or triggers if possible:
- *Symptomatic treatment* with saline, topical intranasal corticosteroids twice daily and oral decongestants as needed.

- Alleviating sympotoms with antihistamines, mucus thinning agents and nasal sprays.
- Thyroid replacement therapy will diminish symptoms associated with hypothyroidism.
- Surgery is useful to correct anatomical abnormalities in the nose and sinuses.
- Treatment of any infection. Prompt and aggressive treatment of infection with antibiotics, along with supplemental medications help to re-establish the normal drainage pathways.
- Restricted diet.

COMMONLY USED MEDICATION

- **Antihistamines** – These drugs block the histamine reaction. They work best when given prior to exposure. Anti-histamines can be divided into two groups:

    1. Sedating (Benadryl, Chlor Trimetron and Tavist).

    2. Non-sedating (Claritin and Hismanal).

- **Decongestants** – These drugs temporarily reduce swelling of sinus and nasal tissues leading to an improvement in breathing and a decrease in obstruction. The most common decongestant is *pseudoephedrine* (Sudafed).
- **Combinations** – These drugs are made up of one or more anti-allergic medications. They are usually a combination of an antihistamine and a decongestant. Other common conbinations include mucus thinning agents, anti-cough agents, aspirin, Advilor Tylenol.
- **Steroid Nasal Sprays** – Vancenase, Beconase, Flonase, Nasacort, Rhinocort. They reduce allergic or inflammatory inflammation, but do not have the side-effect of oral (systemic) steroids.

- **Decongestant Sprays** - (Afrin and Neosynpherine). They quickly reduce swelling of nasal tissues by shrinking the blood vessels.
- **Antihistamine Sprays** - They work like oral antishistamines but applied topically to the nasal membranes (Astelin)
- **Atrovent** - It helps to control nasal drainage mediated by neural pathways. It can decrease nasal drainage.
- **Mucus Thinning Agents** - Mucus thinning agents are utilized to make Secretions more thin and less sticky. Guaifenesin (Humibid, Fenesin) and organic iodine (Organidin) are commonly used formulations.
- **Reflux Medications** - Antacids help to neutralize acid contents, whereas other medication (Tagamen, Peilosec) decrease stomach acid production.

IMMEDIATE ADVANTAGES OF CONVENTIONAL MEDICATIONS

- Decongestants give most consistent relief by shrinking the nasal blood vessels. Some anti-histamines may be helpful when used in combination with decongestants.
- Intranasal corticosteroids are at times helpful in vasomotor rhinitis. Atropine spray can correct part of the overactive intranasal nerve supply and help some people.

DRAWBACKS OF CONVENTIONAL TREATMENT

- Decongestant sprays will improve breathing and drainage over the short term. Unfortunately, if they are used for more than few days they can become highly addictive (rhinitis metamentosa). Long term use can lead to serious damage. Hence, *prolonged use* of over-the-counter nasal decongestant sprays, such as Afrin, will only *worsen* the problem by further irritating the lining of the nose, leading to increased congestion or drainage.

- Often, some people experience nervousness or insomnia, which usually goes away with a miner dosage decrease. Decongestants may aggravate hypertension.
- Symptomatic treatment with saline, topical intranasal corticosteroids twice daily and oral decongestants as needed, may help. But often, these treatments don't work and a patient may start overusing nasal decongestant sprays (i.e. Afrin).
- Anti-histamines are *less effective* in vasomotor rhinitis because histamine is a mediator only in allergic rhinitis.
- Decongestants may also stimulate the action of heart and raise the blood pressure therefore, should be avoided by patients who have high blood pressure, heart irregularity, glaucoma, thyroid problems or difficulty in urination.
- Sedating antihistamines should be avoided in those patients who need to drive or use dangerous equipment. Non-sedating antihistamines can also have serious drug interactions.
- Steroids like *prednisone, medrol, hydrocordisone* etc are highly effective in rhinitis patients, however there is a potential for *serious side effects when used over a period of time.*
- Mucus thinning agents should be discontinued if a rash develops or there is swelling of the salivery glands.

REFERENCES

1. http://www.allergycapital.com.au/Pages/nar.html
2. http://www.medicinenet.com/chronic_rhinitis/page3.htm
3. http://www.aafp.org/afp/20050915.html
4. http://www.regionalallergy.com/vmrinfo.htm

5. http://www.emedicine.com/ent/topic402.htm
6. http://healthcenter.uoregon.edu/patientinfo/allergy_asthma/allergicrhinitis.html
7. http://www.emedicine.com/ent/topic402.htm
8. http://www.allergyclinic.co.nz/guides/50/html

CHAPTER **16**

Homeopathic Perspective of Non-allergic Rhinitis

Naming a disease is not particularly important in homeopathy. Disease label of course can help in indicating the kind of disorder that is affecting the organ or the body. However, symptoms actually do not exist in isolation. They are in fact a reflection of how a person as a whole is coping with his/her reality (stress in life). This also explains why the same disease expresses itself differently in each individual. Hence, the totality of the symptoms experienced by the patient is more important than the name of the disease.

When names of diseases are mentioned, it is always to be understood that the name counts for nothing unless the symptoms are covered with the remedy. If there were no names there would be no routinism, which so often stands in the place of good prescribing.

E. B. Nash[3]

Rhinitis syndrome is a collection of symptoms. Whether allergic or non-allergic it is recognized be the usual symptoms such as sneezing, running nose, lachrymation, itchiness of eye, mouth etc. It is, infact, often difficult to distinguish clinically the non-allergic rhinitis from allergic rhinitis. However, takes into account only the totality of symptoms, whatever may be the name of the disease.

RHINITIS SYNDROMES - FROM HOMEOPATHIC PERSPECTIVE

Dr. H A Roberts comments: "*In considering a case of hay fever, we immediately visualize a syndrome composed of sneezing, lachrymation, red nose, watery coryza.*" He further explains in his essay on hay fever symptoms, "*There is always a hypersensitive state of some one or more of the mucous surfaces: eyes, ears, nose, roof of mouth, uvula tongue, throat, bronchi*". This irritability usually manifests itself in congestion, inflammation, itching, and normally in increased mucus secretions. Occasionally we find the surfaces dry and burning with the congestion, especially if sprays or other local applications of a suppressive nature have been used."

"This hypersensitivity is always *potential* in certain individuals, but it is detonated, as it were, by combinations of predisposing circumstances, such as irritating substances plus favorable thermic, atmospheric and seasonal conditions."

Thus the line-up of remedies is bound to be very similar for both allergic (hay fever) and non-allergic rhinitis Recting in view the similarity of symptoms which overlap significantly.

The Homeopathic treatment begins with a complete analysis *of the patient's symptoms* entire medical history and the patient's personality. This helps in the selection of the homeopathic remedy that is unique to the patient and his/her expression of the rhinitis symptoms. A carefully prescribed remedy kick-starts the healing process which can also eliminate many other health problems.

Hence, treatment of diseas in homeopathy is by comparing the totality of symptoms after forming a picture to picture of medicine.

George Vithoulkas, view in his book "Homeopathy: Medicine of the New Man" this respect is as under:

"When this happens, a phenomenon occurs which is well known to physicists and engineers as "resonance". Just as one tuning fork can stimulate vibration of another of identical frequency, so the remedy enhances the vibration rate of the patient's electomagnetic field. This increases the patient's electromagnetic field at precisely the frequency needed to bring about a cure".

REFERENCES

1. http://www.lifepositive.com/Body/homeopathy/homeopathic-treatment.asp
2. http://www.fishtree.com/whatishomeop.htm
3. E.B. Nash;2002; Leaders in Homoeopathic Therapeutics, Reprint Ed.;B Jain Publishers, New Delhi
4. http://www.homeoint.org/cazalet/roberts/hayfever.htm

CHAPTER 17

Homeopathic Remedies From Different Groups - A Look at the Repertories

REMEDIES FROM DIFFERENT GROUPS

Homeopathic remedies generally fall into the following catagories depending on their *sources:*

i. Botanical Sources:

Flowers, leaves, roots, nuts, seeds and bark etc.

ii. Animal Sources:

Honey bee, insect poisons, snake venoms, spiders ink sprayed by squid etc.

iii. Mineral Sources:

Silver, phosphorus, gold, lead, arsenic, mercury and marble etc.

Remedies from **mineral sources** can be *subdivided* into the further categories:

- Metals – e.g. Cupr. Ferr. Arg.
- Non-Metals – e.g. Sulph; Phos
- Compounds of metals and non metals – e.g. Cupr.ac., Ferr. Phos., Arg. nit., Calc Carb.

iv. **Diseased Tissue:**

Nosodes - e.g. *Psorinum*

v. **Micro-organisms that Cause Diseases:**

Viruses, bacteria etc. e.g. *Influenzinum*

vi. **Radiation:** X-*rays*

vii. **Gases:**

e.g. *Hydrogen* – which is proved by **Dr. Jeremy Sherr.**

viii. **Electricity:** *Electrictas.*

ix. **Magnets – North Pole and South Pole** (*Magnetis polus criticus and australis and etc.*

REMEDIES FOR RHINITIS SYNDROMES

Of the thousands of homeopathic remedies that are available today, those that can potentially alleviate *rhinitis symptoms* may be less than two hundred. It is interesting to note that these remedies come predominantly from plant and mineral sources, and only a few from animal sources and nosodes, as evident from a look at the various repertories.

A LOOK AT THE REPERTORIES

Remedies listed is some of the repertories under the relevant symptoms, mainly sneezing and types of discharge, are given below:

In **Kent's repertory**, we find the following remedies:

SNEEZING

dinner, during :Grat.

      after: Agar., phos., zine.

dry: Ambr., chin., graph.

dust causes: Brom., lyss.

frequent: Acon., agar., *all-c.*, alum., *Am-m.*, ambr., anac., arg-met., am., *Ars.*, asaf., aspar., *aur.*, bar-c., bar-m., *bell.*, *brom.*, *try.*, calc., Carbs., Carb-v., cast., caust., chinin., cic., cist., Coc-c., con., cor-r., crot-h., cupr., *cycl.*, dros., *dulc.*, euph., gins., graph., gymn., *hep.*, kali-ar., *kali-c.*, kali-i., kali-p., kalm., *kreos.*, lact., laur., lil-t., *lyc.*, mag-c., mag-m., mag-s., *Merc.*, mez., mosch., mur-ac., nat-ar., nat-c., nat-m., *nit-ac.*, nux-m., *Nux-v.*, petr., *phos.*, *plan.*, prun-s., ran-s., rhus-t., ruta., *sang.*, sep., sil., spig., *squil.*, stann., staph., *stict.*, stront., *Sulph.*, ther., verat., zinc.

paroxysmal: *Agar.*, arn., bell., calc., con., *gels.*, glon., ham., hell., *ip.*, *kali-i.*, lach., lyss., *nat-m.*, nux-v., phos., *rhus-t.*, sabad., sil., staph., *stram.*, *sulph.*, ther.

walking in open air : Cocc., plat., tarax.

warm room, in : *All-c.*, Puls.

yawning, with : Astac., bry.

Discharge

copious : Acon., aeth., agar., ail., *All-c.*, *alum.*, *alumn.*, anac., anan., *ars-i.*, *Ars.*, arum-t., aspar., bar-c., bar-m., berb., borx., *dry.*, calc-f., calc., canth., carb-s., caust., cedr., chlor., cic., coc-c., coff., cop., cor-r., crot-c., Cupr., *Kali-i.*, lac-c., lact-ac., lyc., mag-m., mur-ac., *nat-ar.*, *nat-c.*, *Nat-m.*, nat-s., *nit-ac.*, nux-v., *Phos.*, plan., plat., *puls.*, rhod., *rumx.*, sabad., *senec.*, sep., *spig.*, *spig.*, staph., *stict.*, *sulph.*, teucr., *tub.*, verat-v., *zinc.*

in open air : Hydr.

from post-nares : Carb-v., Cor–r., euph., *spig.*

with stuffing of head : *Acon.*, agar., arum-t., *calc.*, *Kali.*, *nit-ac.*, *nux-v.*

morning : *Arum-t.*

Boger gives the following :

A SYNOPTIC KEY OF THE MATERIA MEDICA
By CYRUS MAXWELL BOGER

NOSE AND ACCESSORY CAVITIES

Nose and accessory cavities, air, open, amel. :
Aco., All-C., Hydr., Nux-v., Puls., Tell.

Nose and accessory cavities, coryza (fluent discharges):
Aco., Au-c., Ars., Camph., *Cham.*, Euphr., Ferr-p., Gels., Hep., Kali-i., Lach., Merc-c., *Merc.*, Mux-v., *Puls.*, Rhus-t., Sel., Sulph.

Nose and accessory cavities, coryza, annual (hay fever) :
Ambro., *Ars.*, Gels., Kali-i Kali-p., *Nux-v.*, Phos., Sence., Sep., *Sil., Sulph.*

Nose and accessory cavities, coryza, chronic :
Hep., Kali-bi., Sil., Sulph.

Nose and accessory cavities, driping :
An-co., *Ars.*, Arum-t, Calc., Eupipe., Euphr., Graph., Kali-o., Nit-ac., Nex-v., Phos., Sabad., Silp., *Sulph.Tab.*,

Nose and accessory cavities, sneezing :
Ars-i Ars., *Carb-v.*, Cina., *Gels.*, Kali-i., Nat-m., Nux-v., Puls., Rhus-t., Sabad., Sil., *Sulph.*

Nose and accessory cavities, sneezing, abortive :
Carb-v., Sil.

Nose and accessory cavities, sneezing, cough, wigh :
Agar., Gell., Psor., *Squil.*

Nose and accessory cavities, sneezing violent :
Nux-v., Sabad.

Nose and accessory cavities, swelled :
Bell., Cust., Kali-c., Merc., Nat-c., Phos-ac., Puls., Rhus-t., Sep.

Nose and accessory cavities, twitching :
Am-c., *Ambr.,* Aur., *Calc., Chel., Con., Hyos., Kali-bi.,* Nat-m., *Plat.*

Nose and accessory cavities, ulcers :
Ars., Merc., Puls.

Nose and accessory cavities, weather, changing agg. :
Ars.

Nose and accessory cavities, winter, agg. :
Am-c., Ars.Nose and accessory cavities, gushes, fluid : Dulc., Pl-ac., Hydr., Kali-bi., Lach., *Nat-c.,* Nat-m., Phos., Sel., *Thhgic.*

Nose and accessory cavities, polypi :
Cálc., Merc-i-r., Phos., Sang., Thucr.,

Boericke's repertory[4]: Inflammation (rhinitis)

Acute, catarrhal, Pollen irrtation, hay fever, rose cold, summer catarrh – *All.-c., Ambras., Aral., Ars., Ars-i.,* Arum., Arund., Benz-ac., chinin., ars., Cocain., Cupr-ac., Dulc., Eupho-pil., *Euphr.,* Gels., Hep., Hep., Ipec., Kali-i., iod-Kali-s-chrom., *Luch.,* Linu-usit., Merc-i., *Naph.,* Nat., Nat-m., Nux-v., Polla., *Psor.,* Ran-h., Ros-d., *Sabaa.,* Sang., *Sang-n.,* Sil., Sin-n., Skool., Solid., *Stict.,* suprar., Trifp., Tub.

Acute, catarrhal, ordinary cold in head – Acon., AEse., Au-c., Am-c., Am-m., *Ars., Ars-i., Arum-b.,* Avena., Bell., Brom., *Bry., Camph.,* Cham., *Dulc., Eup-Au-c., per-Euphr.,* Ferr-p., *Gels.,* Glyc,Hep., *Hydr.,* Hydr-ac., Iod., *Justi., Kali-gich., Kali-c.,* Lach., Mentho., *Merc-s., Nat-ar., Nat-m., Nux-v.,* Phos., Puls.,*Quill.,* Sabad., Sumb., Sang., *Sang-n.,* Solid., *Stict.,* Ter., Ther., Trom.

CONCOMITANTS

Aching in limbs – Acon., Bry., Eup-per., Gels.

Chilliness (initial stage) – *Acon.,* Bapt., *Camph.,* Caps., Ferr-p., *Gels.,* Merc-i-r., *Nat-m.,* Nux-v., Phyt., *Quill.,* Sapon.

Predisposition to cold – Agra., Alum., Ars., Bac., Bar-c., *Calc.,* Calc-i., Calc-p., Calend., Dulc., Ferr-p., Gels., *Hep.,* Hydr., Kali-c., Merc., *Nat-m.,* Nux-v., Phos., *Psor.,* Sep., Solid., Sulph., Tub.

TYPE OF DISCHARGE IN RHINITIS

Acrid, watery, fluent, hot, or thin mucus – *Au-c., Ambr.,* Am-caust., *Am-m., Aral., Ars.,* Ars-iod., Arum-t., Bell., Carb-v., Cham., Eucal., Gels., Glyc., *Iod., Kali-id.,* Kreos., Lach., *Mer-c.,*Merc., Mur-ac., Naphtin *Nat-h art., Nat-m.,* Nit-ac., *Sabad.,* Sang., Sangin-h.., Sqnil., sulph., Trifx-p.

Albuminous, clear mucus – AEsc., Calc., Camph Graph., Hudr., kali-bi., Kali-i., *Kali-m.,* Lac-c., Menth.,Nat-m., Phos.

Bland mucus – *Euphr.,* Jug-c., *Kali-n* Puls., Sep.

Bloody Mucus – Ail., Arga-n., Ars., *Arum-t.,* Aur., Echi., Hep., Hydr., Kali-Bi., *Merc-l-r.,Pen.,Phos.,* Sangen-n., Sil., Thui.

Green, yellow, fetid (purulent or muco-purulent) -- Alum., Ars., Ars-i., Arum-t., Aur., *Bals-p., Calc.,* Clac-r-i., calc-s., *Dulc.,* Eucal., *Hep., Hydr., Kali-lbi.,*Kali-i., *Kali-s., Lyc.,* Med., *Merc.,* Nat-c., *Nat-s.,* Nit-as., Pen., Phos., *Puls.,* Sung-n., Sep., *Sep.,* Sil., Ther., Thug., Tub.

Membranous formation (See Croupous Rhinitis.) – *Am caust.,* Echi., Hep., *Kali bich.*

Offensive, fetid -- Ars-i., Asaf., *Aur.,* Bals-p., Calc., Echin., Elps., Eucal.,Graph., *Hep., Hydr., Kali-i-bi.,* Kaliiph., Merc-s., Nar-c., Nit-ac., Psor., *Puls.,* Sang., Sep., *Sil., Sul.,* Ther., Tub.

Profuse – Ail., All-c., Am-m., Aral., *Ars., Ars-i., Arum-t.,* Bals-p., Calc-i., *Euphr., Hep., Hydr., Kali-lbi., Kali-i.,* Merc., Nux-v., *Puls.,* Sang., Sangin-n., Sep., Thuj.

Salty-tasting – Aral., Tell.,

Scabs, crusts, plugs – *Alum.,* Arum-sil., Ant-c., Aur-m., Bor-x., Calc-f., Calc-sil., Caust., Elps., Fago., *Graph.,* Hep., *Hydr., Kali-bi.,* Lem-m., *Lyc.,* Merc-i., Nat.,ars., Nit-ac., Petrol., Psor., *puls., Sep.,* Sil., Sticta., Sul., Teict., Ther., Thuya.

Thick – Alum., Am-bro., *Calc.,* Hep., Hydr., *Kali-bi.,* Merc-c., Merc., Nat-c., Pen., *Puls.,* Sep., Ther., Thuj.

Unitateral – Calc-s., Calen., Phyt.

Viscid, ropy, stringy – *Bov.,* Gall-ac., Hydr., Kali-bi., Myrl., Stricta., Sumb.

Itching in nose -- *Agn.,* Au-c., Am-c., Ars-i., *Arund.,* Brom., Cina, Fag., Gly., *Hydr.,* Nat-m., Ram-b., Rosa-d., Sabad., Sang., *Santon-i.,* Sep., Sil., *Teucr., Wye.*

Nervous distubance -- Agar.

Numbness, tingling -- Acon., Jug-c., *Nat-m.,* Plat., Ran-b., Sabad., Sang., Sil., *Stict.*

SNEEZING (Stre nutation) -- Acon., All-c., Am-m., *Aral., Ars.,* Ars-i., Arur.1-t., Arund., Calc., Camph., *Cyel.,* Eupper., Euph., Eu ohr., Gels., Ichth-y., Iod., Kali-bi., *Kali-ac.,* Sang., *Sangin n.,* Sapon., Squil., Sence., Senece., Sebeg., Sin-n., *Stich.*

Chronic tendency --Sil.

Ineffectual -- *Ars.,* Carb-v., Sil.

Coming into warm room : rising from bec :handling peaches -- Au-c.

Cool air, in -- Ars., Hep., Sabad.

Evening, in -- Camph., Caust., Nux-v., Sil.

Immersing hands in water -- Lac-d., Phos.

REFERENCES
1. http://www.fishtree.com/allergies.htm
2. http://www.homeoint.org/books/kentrep1/kent0350.htm#P351
3. http://www.homeoint.org/books2bogersyn/nose.htm

CHAPTER **18**

Treatment of Recurring Allergic/Non-allergic Rhinitis - A Miasmatic Approach

THE IMPORTANCE OF MIASMATIC TREATMENT

The true similimum is always based on the existing miasm and we cannot select the most similar remedy unless we understand the phenomena of the acting miasm. Hence, a knowledge of the underlying principle that causes the manifestations of a clinical disease, becomes necessary in order to monitor the progress of a case.

ANTI-PSORICS TO TREAT RHINITIS SYNDROMES

It is evident from the earlier discussions that the underlying miasm of rhinitis syndromes is psora predominantly. Dr. Hahnemann has postulated that using *anti-psoric medicines to treat the psora miasm would enable to cure effectively.* Hence, any form of rhinitis (allergic, non-allergic or idiopathic), may be effectively treated with deep acting *anti-psoric* remedies.

Based on **Kent's** statement on allergic rhinitis, we may assume that the rhinitis syndrome constitutes *'one of the most difficult conditions to fit a remedy to'.* Symptoms can be palliated easily by short acting remedies, but the cure takes a longer time. *"These symptoms are the outcome of a psoric constitution and must be treated by anti-psorics"* (**Kent**).

For instance, a severe form of rhinitis may seem to be the only manifestation of psora in a patient, but if it is restrained, he may not be well for the whole year. It can be mitigated only by 'constitutional up building'. With careful constitutional treatment, each attack becomes lighter.

According to **H.A.Roberts**, besides the manifestations of the acute diseases, which are all directly traceable to the eruptions of psora, the vital energy often *places the 'psoric poison' in a latent state, where it may lie for a long period, even for years.* Although there may be no manifestations, an "observant physician may read its peculiar characteristics, even in that latent state, and even though the patient is not disturbed to any degree".

Interestingly, this acute manifestation may be due to any one of the various causes. *It may be due to an exposure, or to any other seemingly slight cause.* Whatever may be the direct cause of the acute manifestation, it will show the "poisonous effects" of the miasm, and the physician needs to be conversant with the characteristic of the latent state so that he may "cure the underlying dyscrasia in the latent condition and thus head off the acute manifestations". This would ensure that the resistance power of the vital energy is protected against the sudden strain and help to eradicate the *"psoric poison"*.

A LOOK AT THE ANTI-PSORIC REMEDIES

Some of the **psoric remedies** suggested by **Dr. Hahnemann** include *Sulphur, Natrium mur., Calcarea carb., Arsenic alb., Lycopodium, Phosphorus, Mezereum, Graphites, Causticum, Hepar sulph., Petroleum, Silicea, Zincum met.,* and *Psorinum* amongst many others. "The greatest practical work he did in *Chronic Diseases* was his enlisting the medicines, which were anti-psorics", according to **Dr. Rajendran** in *'The Nucleus - Lectures on Chronic Diseases and Miasms'.*

Keeping the general symptomatology of psoric group, we can take a look at **Boenninghausen's** list of anti-psoric medicines, which comprises of fifty remedies. This list, published in **Hahnemann's** time, has been used with remarkable success in the so-called psoric conditions from that time onwards as seen below:

Agaricus	*Conium*	*Kalicum nit.*
Alumina	*Digitalis*	*Nitricium acid*
Ammonium carb.	*Dulcamara*	*Petroleum*
Ammonium mur.	*Euphorbium*	*Phosphorus*
Anacardium	*Graphics*	*Phosphoricum acid*
Arsenicum alb.	*Guaiaum*	*Platinum*
Aurum	*Hepar sulph.*	*Rhododendron*
Baryta carb.	*Iodicum*	*Sarsaparilla*
Baricum ac.	*Lycopodium*	*Sepia*
Bovista	*Magnesium carb.*	*Silicea*
Calcarea carb.	*Magnesium mur.*	*Stannum*
Carbo animalis	*Manganum*	*Strontium*
Carbo veg.	*Mezereum*	*Sulphur*
Causticum	*Muriaticum acid*	*Sulphuricum acid*
Clematis	*Natrium carb.*	*Zincum*
Colocynth	*Natrium mur.*	

As analysed by **H.A.Roberts**, "Sixteen of the remedies listed (above) belong definitely to the vegetable group, one definitely to the animal group; of the remaining thirty-three remedies, comprising the chemical elements or inorganic substances, or combined from these elements or substances (or reduced to almost elemental consideration, as the *Carbo's*) we find only three (*Baryta, Platinum and Aurum*) *that appear in the range of chemical elements* *higher by atomic weight than those essential to the construction of the human body."*

CHOICE OF ANTI-PSORICS

Peter Morrell[3] has suggested in his article 'Hahnemann's Miasm Theory and Miasm Remedies. *"To discover the **true psoric remedies** we must add together the remedies listed in the repertory for a range of 'psoric' conditions. This means checking carefully all the symptoms and repertorising for all of them, gradually building up a master list of remedies that fit psoric conditions."*

For rhinitis - like symptoms, the following remedies are given by **Kent.** This list includes additional remedies many of which have been ranked as **psoric ++**

S.K. Bannerjee

Rhinitis symptoms (such as hay fever): Ail., All-c., *ars-i., ars., arum-t.,* Arond., bad., *brom., carb-v.,* cycl., *dulc., euphr.,* gels., iod., kali-bi., *kali-p.,* lach., *naja.,* Nat-m., nux-v., Psor., *puls., ran-b.,* Sabad., *sang., sil.,* Sin-n., *stict.,* teucr., *wye.*

Kent p 326

Another indication has been given by **H A Roberts**[6] in his essay on hay fever symptoms: " In an analysis of he results of some ninety cases that have come to us this season, *twelve remedies were indicated and prescribed with satisfactory results,* on the basis of the repertory analysis, in approximately the following proportions:

Pulsatilla, 29% ; Phosphorus, 20% ; Sulphur, 19% ; Nox vomica, 14% ; Sepia, 9% ; Silicea, 51/2% ; Rhus tox, 2% ; Bryonia, 2% ; Calcarea carb., 2%.

Arsenicum album, Sabadilla and Sinapis were prescribed in ne case each, the last not on repertory analysis but on the *obvious indications presented by the patient's symptomatology".*

Some of the remedies often used in the treatment of rhinitis may be represented in the *flow chart* as follows:

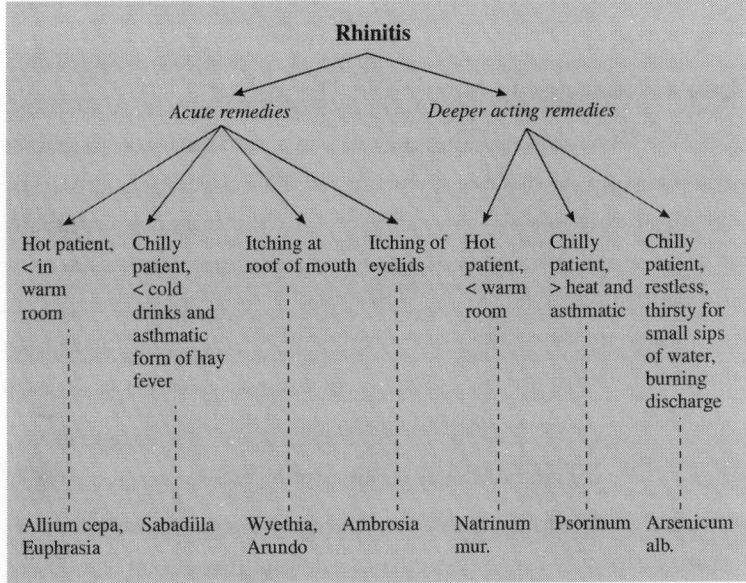

COMMENTS ON SOME MIASMATIC REMEDIES FOR TREATING RHINITIS

For acute management of symptoms, remedies such as Allium cepa, Arundo, Ambrosia, Naphathalinium, and Sabadilla are very useful. For recurring cases, *more deep acting remedies* may be considered such as Natrium mur., Sulphur, Psorinum and Arsenicum, etc. Dr. Nash[7], for instance, recommends Lachesis if paroxysms of sneezing are worse after sleeping, even in day time. *"Lachesis 200 may stop the whole business for the season".*

In *asthmatic forms of rhinitis symptoms* with dyspnea, remedies like Iodum, Arsenicum, Arsenicum iod, Kalium hydr. and Sabadilla are useful. When there is stuffing up of nose not relieved by discharge or blowing. the nose, there is another class of remedies recommended by **Dr. Kent**, which includes *Lachesis,*

Kalium bich, Psorinum, Naja and *Sticta.* The stuffing up of nose is worse in open air but is relieved in a warm room in psorinum whereas *Nux vomica* breathes more easily in open air and his nose gets stuffed up, on entering a warm room.

Use of Nosodes in Miasmatic Treatment

As **Peter Morrell** points out with reference to the use of miasms in treatment, "...many people routinely give the corresponding nosode. For example – a child born with syphilitic skin vesicles, they might give *Syphilinum* rather than the similimum say *Mercurius*. This would tend to be seen as an inappropriate use of the miasm concept, *as the similimum is what the patient needs, not the nosode". The nosode certainly can do good work when it becomes the similimum.*

ROLE OF OTHER MIASMS IN RHINITIS

Dr. Rajendran argues that 'allergic rhinitis does not always mean it is psora'. It can be multi-miasmatic. If sneezing is followed by cold, cough and thick discharge, the miasm will change. *So a prescription has to be the result of "totality made with the concept of miasm".*

Dr. Rajendran emphasizes that there is an implicit relation between miasm and the prescribed drug. He quotes one of his cases of allergic rhinitis where disease tends to progress in every episode, indicating a *tubercular miasm*. This was further confirmed by recurrence and step-by-step development of the disease, which started by sneezing followed by discharge and later by cough and fever. The patient responded well to *Natrium phos.*

According to **Dr. H.A.Roberts,** an *inherited sycotic background* may be responsible for the hay fever or rhinitis symptoms. "Let us ask ourselves why some individuals are immune while others are extremely susceptible. It is true that we occasionally find the hay fever picture actively exhibited in an otherwise apparently healthy person, but upon inquiry we are often able to trace the course of certain suppressions from early childhood *and more than that we usually find an inherited tendency (the stigmatic or miasmatic disease tendencies). Thus we find as the basis for hay fever a background of inheritance usually sycotic, although it may be so far removed from the active stages that we can trace its presence only by the disease tendencies–infiltrative* in nature exhibited at different periods of life."

REFERENCES

1. James Tyler Kent; 2005 *Lectures on Homeopathic Materia Medica*, Reprint Ed.; B Jain Publishers, New Delhi.
2. The Principles and Art of Cure by Homeopathy, H A Roberts, from:
   a. http://www.homeoint.org/books4/roberts/chapter22.htm
   b. http://www.homeoint.org/books4/roberts/chapter24.htm
3. http://www.homeoint.org/morrell/articles/pm_miasm.htm
4. E S Rajendran; 2004; *The Nucleus - Lectures on Chronic Diseases and Miasms*, First Ed.; Mohna Publications, Calicut, Kerala.
5. S K Benerjea; 2005; *Miasmatic Diagnosis*, Reprint Ed.; B Jain Publishers, New Delhi
6. H A Roberts, http://www.homeoint.org./cazalet/roberts/hayfever.htm
7. E B Nash; 2002; *Leaders in Homeopathic Therapeutics*, Reprint Ed.; B Jain Publishers, Niw Delhi
8. http://www.homeoint.org/cazalet/roberts/hayfever.htm

CHAPTER **19**

Important Remedy Profiles in Rhinitis Treatment I - Acute Remedies

"No cure can be made without the similimum; and no case can be analyzed with the Boenninghausen repertory method without the four-square basis of symptoms; the locations, the sensations, the conditions of aggravation and amelioration, and the concomitants."

H.A.Roberts

ACUTE VERSUS CHRONIC REMEDIES

Acute remedies play a very useful role in alleviating the rhinitis symptoms promptly and quickly whereas the underlying chronic cause is addressed only by the deep acting remedies. For instance, **C M Boger** comments on the action of *Sabadilla* on the so-called rose-cold, *"It is very apt to have a palliative action only and it will generally not prevent its yearly recurrence, for which purpose the deeper acting anti-psorics are more suitable."*

Dr. Kent[3] says, while discussing *Sabadilla:* "Many times it will cut short an attack, *but it is not deep acting enough to keep the patient well,* and next season he will have a different kind of coryza and need some other remedy. *This is true of the short acting remedies".*

However, when the patient suffers from a *virulent acute miasm,* *"the treatment of choice is the acute remedy or acute intercurrent".*

In fact, no remedy is exclusively "acute" or exclusively "deep acting" by nature. What is essential is that when the acute state has subsided, the underlying fundamental cause must be removed by *constitutional treatment* to prevent recurrence and complete, the cure.

Discussing the relevance of acute remedies, **David Little** comments Kent in his article: *"A remedy becomes acute or chronic depending on the strategy of the homeopath and how he applies the remedy. Deep acting remedies like Arsenicum, Mercury or Sulphur are often used in acute diseases if the symptoms of the acute layer calls for them. The key in such situations is not to mix the acute and chronic symptoms together in one grand totality as this confuses the case".*

PROFILES OF SOME ACUTE REMEDIES

A wide range of acute remedies are available, *mostly from plant and mineral sources,* and very few from animal sources. Some of the remedies are represented in the *scheme below:*

Some Acute Remedies for Rhinitis Syndromes		
Plant sources	Animal sources	Mineral sources
Ambrosia	Theridion	Arsenicum iod.
Arundo	Apis mel.	Cuperum ac.
Allium cepa	Naja	Natrium ars.
Chininum ars.		Ferrum phos.
Dulcamara		Hepar sulph.
Euphrasia		Kalium sulph.
Rananculus bulb.		Natrium iod.
Sabadilla		Skook ch.
Belladonna		
Sinapis		
Sticta		
Sanguiaria nit.		
Gelsemium		
Arum trip.		
Bryonia		
Ipecacunaha		

These are prescribed, generally in 30C or sometimes in 200C potencies.

Some of the commonly used acute remedies and their characteristics with reference to rhinitis symptoms, are described below.

I. Acute Remedies - From Plant Sources

1. Allium cepa

Family : Liliaceae

For nasal discharge with laryngeal symptoms. 'Specially adapted to phlegmatic patients'. *Allium capa* is indicated by a "bland lachrymation with an acrid coryza, better in the open air and accompanied by sleepiness and flatulency".

Cause, Location and Sensation
- Seasons like spring and autumn; damp winds and while handling peaches
- Eyes, nose, larynx head
- Sensation 'as if hooks were in the larynx or below larynx'; *"as if larynx is split or torn"*
- 'Feeling of a lump at root of the nose'.
- Smarting in eyes as *from smoke,* needs to rub the eyes
- 'Sensation of glowing heat on different parts of the body'

Common symptoms
- Sneezing
- Eyes : burning and smarting, watery and suffused

Characteristic symptoms
- Profuse, acrid, and watery discharge from the nose and bland discharge from eyes (reverse of *Euphraria* which has acrid tears and bland nasal discharge).

Important Remedy Profiles in Rhinitis Treatment I - Acute Remedies

- Acrid discharge dripping from tip of nose *(Ars., Ars-i)*; excoriates lip and wings of nose *(Ars., Arum-p)*
- Nasal discharge lurns and corrodes nose and upper lip.
- *Severe sneezing especially on entering a warm room*; on deep breathing
- *Eyes sensitive to light*
- Dull headache < in evening, warm room *(Euphr.)*; > in open air *(Puls.)*
- Very sensitive to odor of flowers and *skin of peaches*
- Every year in August *(Naja)*, morning coryza on rising from bed, with violent sneezing

Modalities
- < in evening, warm room *(Euphr.)*
- > in cold room and open air *(Puls.)*

Associated symptoms Relationship
- Laryngeal symptoms; hoarseness; tendency to nasal polyps. Complements Puls. and Phos.
- Similar to *Euphrasia*, but lachrymation and coryza are opposite.

2. Sabadilla
Family : Liliacea

Has special action on mucous membrane of nose and lachrymal glands producing symptoms like hay fever. Good for asthmatic form of hay fever; 'suitable for people with weak and relaxed muscular system'.

Sabadilla is characterized by repeated fits of sneezing, sometimes up to 10 sneezes in a row, and a nose that "runs like a tap." There is extreme sensitivity to odors, especially fragrances. In rhinitis, it is indicated by the *predominant sneezing*, with itching and tingling within the nose, complete obstruction and a watery discharge, all worse in the open air.

C M Boger points out that in this disease, "it merits comparison with *Allium cepa, Squilla, Arundo, Wyethia, Nux vomica* and *Kalium bichromicum.*" It is particularly helpful in wormy children who have snuffles. In general, the symptoms predominate on the right side or go from thence to the left. In the throat however, the reverse holds good.

Cause
- Flowers; odor of flowers, fruits and other smells.
- Seasons like spring or autumn.

Location
- Eyes, nose, throat and head

Sensation
- Sensation of skin hanging loosely in throat, must swallow over it
- Sensation of lump in throat with *constant desire to swallow*
- Sensation of great rawness in the nose

Common symptoms
- Eyelids red and burning, lachrymation; sneezing and coryza
- Stuffed up nostrils with labored inspirations and itching in the nose
- Face feels hot; severe frontal pains and headache

Characteristic symptoms
- *Oversensitive to odors of flowers,* fruits, or garlic "Even thinking of odor of flowers makes him sneeze". (*Sanguinaria* sensitive to flowers).

- Stitches, soreness and pain in throat which goes from left to right (*Lach., Lac-c.*)
- *Violent* sneezing in *spasmodic paroxysms,* followed by lachrymation
- Copious watery nasal discharge with thin mucus at first, later thick mucus
- Dyspnea, asthmatic form of hay fever
- Can swallow warm foods more easily (reverse of *Lach* < by warm food and relieved by cold food); empty swallowing is more painful.
- Chilly patient - sensitive to cold air; cold room and cold food.

Modalities
- < by cold and cold drinks; odor of flowers; full moon/ new moon
- > *by warm food and water* (*Lyc.*) by inhaling hot air; wrapped up; in open air (*Puls.*)

Associated symptoms
- Dysphagia; dyspnea; tendency to asthmatic form of hay fever; parchment-like dryness of skin; *worm affections in children* (*Cina, Sil.*)

Mind
- Timid; nervous; *illusion that she is very sick and 'has some horrible throat disease that is fatal'*

Relationship
- Complements *Sepia.*
- Comparable to *Arsenicum* especially in the respiratory sphere, according or **C M Boger.**

3. Squilla maritima (Sea onion)

A slow acting remedy. It acts especially on the mucous membranes of the respiratory and digestive tracts. "This remedy is needed if there is much bloating around the eyes, while the patient continually rubs them and sneezes", according to C M Boger. The teeth may show back marks. The tincture is prepared using the fresh bulb.

Cause
- Irritants; allergens; change from warm to cold air and cold drinks

Location
- Eyes, nose and throat

Sensation
- Sensation in eyes - as if swimming in cold water
- Margin of nostrils feel sore
- Icy coldness of hands and feet

Common symptoms
- Sneezing and coryza.

Characteristic symptoms
- Eyes feel irritable - child rubs them with fists
- Fluent coryza; sneezing; copious, colorless flow from the nose, especially in the morning
- Violent sneezing; nasal discharge acrid and corroding; < in morning
- Throat irritated; cough provoked by taking deep breath or cold drinks
- Involuntary spurting of urine and sneezing; child rubs face with fist during cough (Caust., Puls.)

Important Remedy Profiles in Rhinitis Treatment I - Acute Remedies

- Copious and acrid flow of mucus and burning (Ars.)
- Constant desire to swallow saliva; difficulty in swallowing
- Chilly patient; can not have the least draft; very sensitive to cold

Modalities
- < by motion
- > rest

Associated symptoms
- Dyspnea; dull rheumatic pains

Relationship
- Squilla follows Digitalis well

4. Wyethia helenioides (Poison weed)

Has marked effects on throat and hay fever symptoms, especially in autumn. According to **Dr. Kent**, *"Wyethia will cure for the season, and it has cured permanently in some cases."*

Cause
- Autumn; allergens

Location
- Eyes, nose and throat

Sensation
- Lips and mouth feel as if scalded
- Itching in the palate and posterior nares
- Dry sensation in throat although mucus is abundant
- Sensation of heat down esophagus
- Tickling on the edges of eyelids

Common symptoms
- Sneezing and coryza

Characteristic symptoms
- Itching of the soft palate, in the roof of the mouth; compelled to scratch it with the tongue (Arundo)
- Extreme dryness of mucous membranes of nose, mouth and throat, although mucus is abundant
- Copious and acrid flow of mucus with burning (*Ars.*)
- Constant desire to swallow saliva; difficult swallowing

Modalities
- < in the afternoon

Associated symptoms
- Tendency to get hoarse while talking or singing dry asthma and hemorrhoids

Mind
- Great depression of spirits, nervous and uneasy

Gelsemium *(Yellow Jasmine)*
Family : Loganiaceae

Acts on the nervous system - complete relaxation and prostration of whole muscular system with entire motor paralysis. "In lingering acute troubles.... it is very useful, but in chronic miasms it is not the remedy. It is only a short acting remedy, though slow in its beginning." - **Dr. Kent.**

Cause
- Bad effects from fright, fear, exciting news and sudden motions (*Ign.*- from pleasant surprise, *Coff.*); irritants; allergens.

Location
- Eyes, nose, throated head

Sensation
- Sensation in eyes, *eyelids feel heavy*
- head feels heavy with a *sensation of a band around the head above eyes* (*Carb-ac., Sulph*).
- Feeling of lump in the throat that cannot be swallowed.
- Itching and tickling in soft palate and naso-phrynx.

Common symptoms
- Sneezing and coryza

Characteristic symptoms
- Eyes feel heavy drooping eyelids patient can hardly open them.
- Sneezing; fullness at the root of the nose
- Acute coryza with dull headache; fever
- Face is hot, flushed and besotted-looking (Bapt., Op.)
- Difficult swallowing; pain in the ear on swallowing (*Hep., Nux-v.*)
- Chilly patient

Modalities
- < damp weather; emotions excitement, bad news, tobacco smoke, thinking of his ailment, before a thunder storm.
- Bending forward, profuse urination, open air, continued motion and stimulants.

Associated symptoms
- Aphonia; lack of thirst; oppression about the chest

Mind
- Desires to be left alone; dull; listless; fear of death (*Ars.*); lack of self-confidence and courage. Anticipatory anxiety in the face of any ordeal, meeting, engagement; etc.; stage fright, nervous dread of appearing in public (*Arg-n.*).

Relationship
- Antidoted by *China, Coffea*.

6. Dulcamara
Common name: Bitter-sweet
Family : Solanaceae

Adapted to persons of phlegmatic scrofulous constitution; restless, irritable. Constitutional state "disturbed by every change in the weather, from warm to cold, from dry to moist, and from suddenly cooling the body while perspiring." - **Dr. Kent**.

Cause
- Exposure to cold, damp, rainy weather, or sudden changes in hot weather (*Bry.*), living or working in cold basement, (*Nat-s.*); sitting on cold damp ground.

Location
- Eyes, nose, throat and head.

Sensation
- Icy coldness; wants nose to be kept warm.
- Eyes feel sore; "every time he takes a cold, it settles in the eyes".

Common symptoms
- Eyes sore and red, lachrymation; coryza.
- Stuffed up nose; Itching in nose; sneezing.
- Headache.

Characteristic symptoms

- Very sensitive to newly grown grass and drying weeds.
- Increased secretion from mucous membranes. while the skin is inactive.
- Profuse discharge of water from nose and eyes < in open air; > in closed room, on waking up in the morning.
- Complete stoppage of nose; patient may have to sleep with mouth open.
- Nose stuffs up when there is a cold rain; constant sneezing; cannot breathe through nose (*Lach.*).
- Wants nose to be kept warm, least cold air stops the nose.
- Thick yellow mucus from nose.
- Eyes swelled and most affected; then nose; then again eyes; granular lids; profuse watery duscharge, < in open air.
- Congestive headache.
- Hay fever.
- Chilly patient, sensitive to cold air.

Modalities

- < By cold and cold air; cold wet weather; sweat; suppressed menstruation; at night.
- > By moving about (*Rhus tox., Ferr.*), external warmth; dry weather.

Associated symptoms

- Skin eruptions, especially urticaria; catarrhal rheumatism; warts, fleshy, large and smooth on face, back of hands and fingers (*Thuja*).

Mind
- Mental confusion; cannot find the right word for anything.

Relationship
- Complementary to, *Baryta carb., Kali-s.*
- Incompatible with, *Bell., Lach.,* should not be used before or after.
- Follows well after, *Cal., Bry., Lyc., Rhus-t., Sep.*

7. Arundo mauritanica (Weed)

Arundo, as pointed out by **Dr. Allen,** is perhaps one of the most important remedies for this disorder. It is a remedy for catarrhal states. Itching is the most outstanding feature relieved by Arundo.

Dr. Kent gives this drug in black type in the repertory for hay fever.

There is *intense itching of the eyes, nose, insides of the ears and particularly the roof of the mouth* (*Wyethia*). *There can be sneezing* (*not in fits like Sabadilla*) *as well as a loss of sense of smell* (*Nat-m.*).

Cause
- Irritants; allergens.

Location
- Eyes, nose palate.

Sensation
- Burning and itching in the palate and conjunctiva.
- Itching of nostrils and roof of the mouth.

Common symptoms
- Sneezing; coryza; headche.

Characteristic symptoms
- Itching of the soft palate, in the roof of the mouth (Wyethia).
- Annoying itch in the nostrils and the roof of the mouth, with sneezing.
- With sneezing, pieces of indurated greenish mucus.
- Running of frothy mucus from the nose; first water dischage, later green mucus form nose.
- Itching, burning, dryness of Schneiderian membrane
- Coryza; loss of smell (*Nat-m.,*)
- Deep seated pain in the sides of the head.

Associated symptoms
- Dyspnea; longing for acids.

8. Euphrasia officinalis

Common Name: Eyebright

Family: Scrophularaceae

Good remedy for catarrhal affections of mucous membranes, especially of the eyes and nose.

Cause
- Irritants; allergens.

Location
- Eyes, nose, throat.

Sensation
- Burning lachrymation; gritty feeling in eyes.
- Burning in the margin of eye lids.

Common symptoms
- Sneezing; lachrymation; coryza

Characteristic symptoms
- Profuse, acrid lachrymation, with profuse, bland coryza (reverse of *All-c.*).
- The eyes water all the time and are agglutinated in the morning.
- Margins of lids red, swollen, burning. Frequent inclination to blink.
- Profuse fluent coryza in morning with violent cough and abundant expectoration, <from exposure to warm south wind.
- Excessive lachrymation during cough.
- Sticky mucus on cornea; must wink to remove it.
- Cough only in day time (*Fer., Nat-m.*).

Modalities
- < In the evening, in bed, indoors, warmth, moisture, after exposure to south wind, when touched (*Hep.*).
- > Coffee; in dark

Associated symptoms
- Amenorrhea, with catarrhal symptoms of eyes and nose; frequent yawning when walking in open air.

Relationship
- Similar to *Puls.* in affections of the eyes; reverse of *All-c.*, in lachrymation and coryza.
- Antidoted by *Camphora* and *Puls.*

9. Sinapis Nigra

Common name: Black mustard

The remedy is useful in hay fever symptoms, coryza and pharyngitis. It is characterized by the stoppage of alternate nostrils and acanty, acrid discharge.

Important Remedy Profiles in Rhinitis Treatment I - Acute Remedies

Cause
- Irritants; allergens.

Location
- Eyes, nose, pharynx.

Sensation
- Mucus from posterior nares feels cold.
- Throat feels scalded.
- Smarting in the eyes.

Common symptoms
- Sneezing; coryza; lachrymation.

Characteristic symptoms
- Stoppage of left nostril all day or in afternoon and evening.
- Mucous membrane of nose dry and hot.
- *Nostrils alternately stopped.*
- Nose swollen and stuffed.
- Dryness of anterior nares.
- Thin, acrid discharge (*Ailanthus*).
- Eyes suffused, itching, smarting.
- Lachrymation with sneezing.

Modalities
- < In afternoon or evening
- > Cough relieved by lying down

Associated symptoms
- Sweat on upper lip and forehead.

Relationship
- Similar to *Sinapis alba* (white mustard) in throat symptoms.

II. Acute Remedies From Mineral Sources

10. Ferrum phosphoricum

Common name: Phosphate of Iron – $Fe_2[PO_4]_3$

Useful in the first stage of inflammatory affections, especially for catarrhal affections of respiratory tract.

Cause
- Irritants; allergens.

Location
- Eyes, nose, pharynx.

Sensation
- Burning sensation in the eyes.
- Feeling as if sand under lids.

Common symptoms
- Coryza; headache.

Characteristic symptoms
- Eyes red, with burning sensation.
- Predisposition to colds; epistaxis.
- Flushed face.
- Fauces red, inflamed; sore throat.
- Hoarseness; short tickling cough.

Modalities
- < At night 4 - 6 a.m.; touch; jar; motion.
- > Cold application.

Important Remedy Profiles in Rhinitis Treatment I - Acute Remedies

Associated symptoms
- Anemic with false plethora and eyes flushing.

Mind
- Nervous, sensitive.

Relationship
- Comparable to *Aconitium, Gelsimium*.
- China for febrile conditions.

11. Cuprum aceticum
Common name: Acetate of copper - Cu $[CH_3COO]_2$

Cause
- Irritants; allergens.

Location
- Nose, head, throat.

Sensation
- Heaviness of head.
- Burning, stinging in temples and forehead.

Common symptoms
- Hay fever; headache.

Characteristic symptoms
- Tough, tenacious mucus; fears suffocation.
- Burning excoriation.
- Paroxysmal cough.
- Constant protrusion and retraction of tongue (*Lachesis*).
- Neuralgia with heaviness of head.
- Head reels in high-ceiled room.

Modalities
- < Mental emotions; touch.

- > Chewing; pressure; at night; warmth; lying on the affected side.

Associated symptoms
- Head reels when in high-ceiled room.

Mind
- Fear of suffocation; inclined to gape and cry.

Relationship
- Acts similarly to *Cuprum met.*, but is more violent in action.

III. Acute Remedies From Animal Sources

12. Naja tripudians

Common name: Cobra

Family: Elapidae

Naja is one of the remedies indicated by **Dr. Margaret L Tyler** in *"Pointers to Some Hay fever Remedies"*. Suffocative attacks in August (*Allium cepa*). Like *Lach.* wakes suffocating, gasping, choking.

Cause
- Irritants; allergens.

Location
- Nose, throat, head.

Sensation
- *Sense of choking;* grasps at throat.
- Larynx and trachea feel raw.
- Feeling of weight over heat.

Common symptoms
- Sneezing; runny nose; hay fever.

Characteristic symptoms
- *Dry larynx.*
- Much sneezing; can not lie down at night.
- Rawness of trachea and larynx, *as if excoriated.*
- Eyes staring; ptosis of both lids.
- Sticky mucus and saliva.
- Irritating dry cough.
- *Gasping at throat* with sense of choking.

Modalities
- < From use of stimulants.
- > From walking or riding in open air.

Associated symptoms
- Dyspnea; asthma beginning with coryza.

Mind
- Broods constantly over imaginary troubles; depressed; dreads to be left alone.

Relationship
- Comparable to other snake remedies like *Lachesis* in suffocating attacks.

REFERENCES
1. http://www.homeoint.org/cazalet/roberts/hayfever.htm
2. http://www.homeoint.org/cazalet/boger/sabadilla.htm
3. http://www.homeoint.org/cazalet/kent/sabadilla.htm
4. http://www.simillimum.com/Thelittlelibrary/Casemanage/kentonacutes.html
5. H C Allen; 2004; *Allen's Keynotes - Rearranged and Classified*, Reprint Ed.; B Jain Publishers, New Delhi.

6. William Boericke; 2003; *Homoeopathic Materia Medica, and Repertory,* Reprint Ed.; B Jain Publishers, New Delhi.
7. James Tyler Kent; 2005; *Lectures on Homoeopathic Materia Medica,* Reprint Ed.; B Jain Publishers, New Delhi.
8. http://www.homeoint. org/cazalet/tyler/hayfever.htm
9. http://www.alive.com/896a3a2.php?subject_bread_cramb=227
10. Pictures from http://images.google.com/sg/imghp?hl=en

CHAPTER **20**

Important Remedy Profiles in Rhinitis Treatment II - Deep Acting Remedies

"Prescrible for the patient first. No results of disease should be removed until proper constitutional treatment has been resorted to, and be sure that it is proper....."

Dr. J.T. Kent. (Lectures on Homeopathic Materia Medica)

THE ROLE OF DEEP ACTING REMEDIES

Although the short acting remedies meet the symptomatic indications of rhinitis symptomatic, they do not meet the 'needs of the patient as a whole'. To treat the underlying cause, a deep acting or a constitutional remedy is required. For instance, **Dr. H. A. Roberts** remarks on treating hay fever, *"In the case where Sinapis was used so successfully, this was the complementary remedy to Sulphut in this case, for Sulphur had been to constitutional remedy and had released the effects of early suppressed eruptions........We cannot possibly consider any case until and unless we have removed the hypersensitivity to material activating ittitants."*

CHOICE OF REMEDIES

Hence, treating the patient rather than the syndrome actually cures the tendency by correcting the constitutional basis and restoring the state of health. While giving directions for forming a *'Complete image of a disease'*, **Dr. B.C. von**

Boenninghausen writes:

> "For it is not only taught by experienc, but it lies in the nature of all chronic diseases which have in consequence been interwoven with the whole organism, that rarely or never one remedy will cover the whole complex of symptoms; so that it will be necessary in order to destory the whole malady fundamentally to let several medicines, selected after each report, operate, until nothing morbid may be left."

As seen earlier, remedies such as *Sabadilla, Allium cepa*, etc. are very useful for managing the acute symptoms of rhinitis. For recurring cases, constitutional or deep acting miasmatic remedies may be selected such as *Tuberculinum, Thuja, Sulphur*, etc. based on the *totality of symptoms*. (For instance, *Lachesis* is recommended by **Dr. Nash**, if paroxysms of sneezing are worse after sleeping, even in day time.)

Another set of remedies such a *Kalium bich., Psorinum*, etc. are useful when a stuffy nose is not relieved by discharge or blowing the nose. Modalities play an important role as well. For instance, the *Nux vomica* nose gets stuffed up on entering a warm room whereas the *Psorinum* nose is relieved in a warm room. Remedies such as *Arsencum iod.* and *Kalium hydn.* are indicated in asthmatic forms of rhinitis with dyspnea.

Deep Acting Remedies From Different Groups

A number of deep acting and/or constitutional remedies are available from different sources including plant, animals, minerals and nosodes. The flow chart below shows some of these remedies

Important Remedy Profiles in Rhinitis Treatment II- Deep Acting Remedies

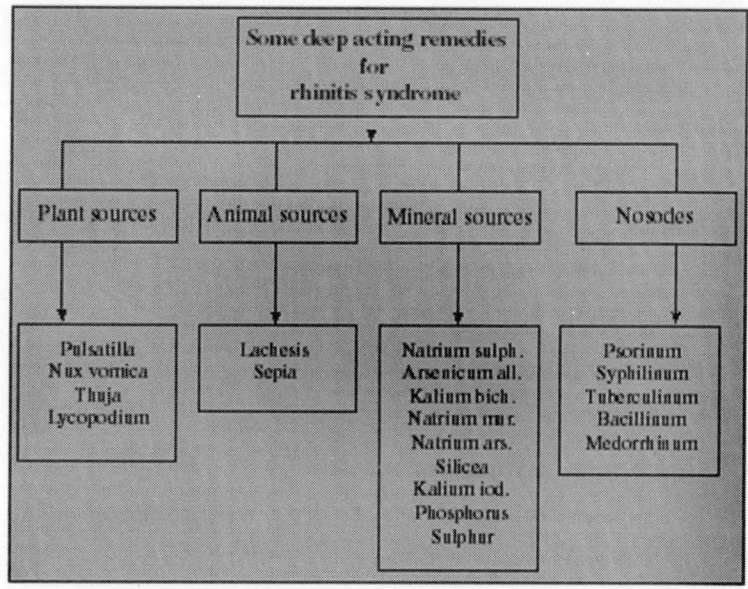

These are prescribed in 30 or 200C to 1M potencies and also in *LM potencies*, whenever necessary.

PROFILES OF SOME DEEP ACTING REMEDIES

A few of these deep acting and/or constitutional remedies and their characteristics with reference to rhinitis symptoms are described below:

I. Deep Acting Remedies - From Plant Sources

1. Pulsatilla nigricans

Common name : Wind flower

Family : Ranunculaceae

A good remedy to start the treatment in chronic cases (*Sulph., Cal.*), Anti-sycotic as well as anti-psoric remedy. The disposition and mental stante are the chief guiding symptoms for the selection of Pulsatilla. Also useful when there is a bacterial or secondary infection in the respiratory tract.

Cause
- Irritants; allergens.

Location
- Eyes, nose, pharynx.

Sensation
- Itching and burning in eyes.
- Itching at the roof of mouth at night.

Common symptoms
- Sneezing; coryza; lachrymation.

Characteristic symptoms
- Nasal discharge during the day and congestion at night.
- Profuse yellowish green mucus; purulent expectoration.
- Loss of smell; stoppage of right nostril.
- Headache in the forehead.
- Profuse lachrymation.
- Ever changing symptoms.
- Chilly patient, but seeks open air and feels better there.

Modalities
- < Twilight aggravation; warm room; hot weather; rich food; while lying down.
- > Cool rooms; open air; cold applications; cold food and drinks

Associated symptoms
- *Lack of thirst;* involuntary uritation with cough (*Caust.*).

Mind
- Gently, yielding disposition; tendency to weep; desires sympathy.

Relationship
- Complementary to *Coffea, Chamomilla, Nux vomica*.
- Chronic of *Pulsatilla* is *Silicea*.

2. Thuja occidentalis (Coniferae)

Thuja is the *'King of anti-sycotic'*, remedies and is well known for its action on skin, especially figwarts and condylomata. It is suitable for people with dark complexion and hydrogenoid constitutions.

Cause
- Irritants; allergens; ill effects of vaccination; maltreated gonorrhea (*Med.*).

Location
- Eyes, nose, pharynx.

Sensation
- Painful pressure at root of nose.
- Eyes feel as if a cold stream of air is blowing.

Common symptoms
- Sneezing; coryza.

Characteristic symptoms
- Chronic catarrh; thick green mucus.
- Dryness of nasal cavities.
- Pain at the root of nose.
- On blowing nose, a pressing pain in teeth (Boenninghausen).
- Chilly patient, left sided.

Modalities
- < Damp, humid atmosphere; at night; after breakfast; vaccination.

- > Dry weather; left side; drawing up a lim.

Associated symptoms
- Constipation or diarrhea; anal fissures; nails are brittle and deformed.

Mind
- Constantly in a hurry; quarrelsome; fixed ideas (for instance, "as if something alive in the abdomen"); music causes weeping.

Relationship
- Complementary to *Arsenicum*, *Silicea*, *Natrium sulph*.

II. Deep Acting Remedies - From Mineral Sources

3. Sulphur

A great Hahnemannian anti-psoric with "centrifugal action – from within outward". Very useful when carefully selected remedies fail to act. Sulphur can arouse the 'reactionary powers' of the organism and is of great use in the beginning of treatment of chronic cases and for complaints that relapse.

Cause
- Irritants; allergens.

Location
- Eyes, nose pharynx.

Sensation
- Burning in the eyes.
- Pressure as from a lump in throat; ball seems to rise and close the pharynx.

Common symptoms
- Sneezing; coryza; itching; headache.

Characteristic symptoms
- Heat and burning in eyes (*Ars., Bell.*).
- Nose stuffed indoors; fluent nasal discharge outdoors.
- Burning nasal discharge.
- Burning, redness and dryness of throat.
- Oppression and burning sensation in chest.
- Dyspnea in middle of night, relieved by sitting up.

Modalities
- < At rest; when standing; warmth of bed; bathing; in morning; 11 a.m.
- > Dry warm weather.

Associated symptoms
- Redness of orifices; sinking feeling in stomach at 11 a.m.; dislike for water.

Mind
- Irritable, depressed; forgetful; lazy, children dislike bathing.

Relationship
- *Sulphur* is the chronic of *Aconitum* and complementary to *Psorinum*.
- *Sulphur* is followed well by *Calcarea* and *Lycopodium* in the given order.
- *Calclarea* should not be used before *Sulphur*.

4. Natrium muriatium
Common name : Common salt (NaCl)

Deep acting and long acting remedy which can make 'lasting changes; by treading the underlying susceptibility to periodic attacks. Great sensitivity for 'colds that commence with sneezing'.

Some patients may develop their symptoms after an emotional experience, especially after grief. Any emotional trauma such as death, divorce, unrequited love, or homesickness can create deep-rooted feelings that are not fully expressed, eventually leaking to various physical complaints, for which Natrium mur. is an effective remedy.

Cause
- Exposure to any allergen or irritant.

Location
- Eyes, nose, head, throat.

Sensation
- Squirming sensation in nostril, as of a small worm, pain like 'thousand little hammers in head knocking on the brain'.

Common symptoms
- Sneezing; lachrymation; coryza.

Characteristic symptoms
- Characteristic nasal discharge; with and watery 'like raw white of an egg'.
- Loss of smell and taste; violent sneezing.
- Lachrymation burning and acrid; eyelids swollen.
- *Fluent coryza changes into stopped nose after 1-3 days, making breathing difficult;* internal soreness of nose.
- Throbbing headache on awakening and from sunrise to sunset.

Modalities
- < In warm room (*Allium cepa*); morning 10 or 11 a.m. (< evening, *Puls.*); music; lying down; at sea-shores
- > In open air (*Puls.*); tight clothing.

Associated symptoms
- Frontal sinus; tendency to periodic headaches and constipation.

Mind
- Irritable, depressed and brooding; *consolation aggravates.*

Relationship
- Complements *Apis* and acts well before or after it.
- Followed well by *Sepia*.

5. Arsericum album
Common name : White oxide of arsenic - As_2O_3

A proven remedy in the treatment of nasal allergies and good for "complaints that return annually" (*Carb-v., Lach., Sulph*). Sneezing is a prominent symptom - starts from tickling in one spot in the nose; after sneezing, tickling is as bad as before

(Dr Margaret L. Tyler[5])

Cause
- Exposure to allergens or irritants.

Location
- Eyes, nose, throat.
- Feeling of *burning* in eyes, nose and throat.

Common symptoms
- Lachrymation; sneezing; coryza.

Characteristic symptoms
- Thin, watery discharge, burning and excoriating.
- Discharge burns a red streak over the upper lip and about the wings of nose.
- Sneezing without relief; nose feels stopped up; < in open air (*Puls.* - better in open air); > indoors.

- Burning in eyes with acrid lachrymation.
- Dyspnea (*Sabad., Ars-i.*); unable to lie down; fears suffocation.
- Great thirst for small quantities of water.
- Great exhaustion after the slightest exertion.

Modalities
- < midnight; cold drinks; wet weather; sea-shore (*Nat-m.*).
- > Indoors; heat (reverse of *Euphr., Sec.*); warm drinks (*Sabad. Lyc.*).

Associated symptoms
- Dyspnea; can not bear the sight or smell of food.

Mind
- *Restlessness; changes place continually; anguish; fears.*

Relationship
- Complementary to *Carb-v.* and *Rhus-t.*
- Compares with *Nat-m.* and *Aqua marina* for sea-side complaints.

III. Deep Acting Remedies - From Animal Sources

6. Lachesis muta
Common name: Surukuku snake
Family: Ophidia

Lachesis is a frequently indicated remedy and *"seems to fit the whole human race"* according to **Dr. Kent**. The catarrhal symptoms of nose are prominent with stuffing up of nose, over-sensitiveness to odors and chronic inflammatory canditions.

Cause
- Irritants; allergens; ill effects of suppressed discharges;

long lasting grief, fright, jealousy, etc. (*Aur., Ign., Ph-ac.*).

Location
- Eyes, nose and pharynx

Sensation
- Dry stuffed sensation through head
- Sore nostrils and lips; sensation of suffocation *when anything is around throat*
- Sensation as if eyes were drawn together by cords tied in a knot at the root at the nose

Common symptoms
- Sneezing; coryza; headache

Characteristic symptoms
- Paroxysms of sneezing (*Silicea; Sabad.*), worse after sleep even in the day time
- Mucus membrane or nose thickened
- Watery discharge from nose may alternate with catarrhal headaches
- *Throat sensitive to touch or pressure; can not swallow warm drinks*
- Face red, puffed
- Eyes seem almost pressed out
- Headache extending into nose, with violent paroxysms of sneezing
- *Sleeps into aggravation; oversensitive to touch and noise*

Modalities
- < After sleep (*Kali-bich.*); left side; pressure or constriction; warm bath; hot drinks

- Warm applications; appearance of discharges

Associated symptoms
- Hemorrhagic tendency; can not bear anything tight anywhere

Mind
- Suspicious; jealous; great loquacity; restless and uneasy

Relationship
- Followed well by - *Crotalus*
- Complementary - *Lyc., Hep.*
- Incompatible - *Acet-ac., Carb-a.* Antidoted by *Ars., Merc.*

7. Sepia
Comman name : Cuttle fish
Family : Mollusca

"Sepia has a marked catarrhal tendency to milky discharges from mucus membranes," with prolonged catarrh of nose and thick greenish-yellow mucus.

Cause
- Irritants; allergens

Location
- Eyes, nose, pharynx

Sensation
- Chest feels opressed
- Sensation of lump in throat (*Lachesis*)

Common symptoms
- Sneezing; coryza; headache

Characteristic symptoms
- Cough with profuse expectoration
- Thick, green discharge
- Thick yellowish crusts fill the nose and cannot be blown out
- Pain at the root of nose
- Chronic nasal catarrh, especially post-nasal
- Chilly patient; feels cold even in a warm room

Modalities
- < Washing; laundry work; dampness; before thunderstorm
- > Exercise; pressure; hot applications; warmth of bed; after sleep

Associated symptoms
- Dyspnea; yellow or brownish saddle across the nose and cheeks

Mind
- Indifferent to loved ones; averse to occupation; weeps while telling symptoms

Relationship
- Complementary to *Nat-m. Phos., Nux-v.*
- Followed well by *Guaiacum*

IV. Deep Acting Remedies - Nosodes

8. Psorinum

"Hay fever appearing regularly every year at the same day of the month" **Kent**. Useful for patients with *Psoric, eczematous and asthmatic history*. "Patient should be treated in the previous winter to eradicate the diathesis and prevent the summer attack." *Psorinum is useful when well-selected remedies fail to act.* It can be given in 200C as an intercurrent remedy.

P. B. Bell: *"Whether derived from purest gold or purest filth, our gratitude for its excellent service forbids us to inquire or care."*

Cause
- Irritants; allergens; fall season every year; *suppressed skin eruptions*
- Eyes, nose, head
- Feeling of ulceration in cornea and under the sternum, throat may feel scalded and burning

Common symptoms
- Inflamed eyelids; coryza; stuffed nose

Characteristic symptoms
- Photophobia with inflamed lids, eyes agglutinated
- Stuffing up of the nose in the fall
- There is some *dyspnea* which is relieved by lying down and stretching the arms at right angles to the body (reverse of *Ars.*)
- Nose dries up part of the time; *must blow the nose all the time in early stages*
- Coryza with thick yellowish-green discharge (*Puls.*)
- Dropping from posterior nares
- Secretions have a filthy smell
- Chilly patient *extremely* sensitive to cold

Modalities
- < Coffee (*Ignatia*), changes of weather, least cold air, open air
- \> Heat (reverse of *Euphr.*), lying down, warm *clothing even in summer*

Associated symptoms
- Dyspnea; sweating; tendency to skin symptoms and

asthma; debility
Mind
- Nervous, restless, anxious, hopeless, despairs of recovery

Relationship
- Complementary to *Sulphur* and *Tuberculinum*
- Followed well by *Sulphur*

9. Tuberculinum

Adapted to persons of tubercular diathesis. *Useful when there is family history of tubercular affections and the best selected remedy fails to give relief or cure. Adapted to persons of tubercualr diathesis. Good remedy for recurrent conditions.*

Cause
- Irritants; allergens

Location
- Eyes, nose, pharynx

Sensation
- Intense headache, as if an iron band around the head
- Sensation of suffocation even with plenty of fresh air

Common symptoms
- Sneezing; coryza; headache

Characteristic symptoms
- Thick expectoration
- Sense of suffocation; longs for cold air
- Disposition *to take cold easily on the slightest exposure*
- Symptoms ever changing

- Loss of weight

Modalities
- < Motion; music; before a storm; dampness; early morning
- > Open air

Associated symptoms
- Pronounced emaciation while eating well (*Nat-m.*)

Mind
- Melancholy, despondent; irritable; fear of dogs; everything in the room seems strange.

Relationship
- Follows *Psorinum* well in hay fever symptoms.
- Complementary to *Sulphur.*

REFERENCES

1. James Tyler Kent; 2005; *Lectures on Homoeopathic Materia Medica*, Reprint Ed.; B Jain Publishers, New Delhi.
2. http://www.homeoint.org/cazalet/roberts/hayfever.htm
3. http://www.homeoint.org/cazalet/boenninghausen/image.htm
4. E B Nash; 2002; *Leaders in Homoeopathic Therapeutics*, Reprint Ed.; B Jain Publishers, New Delhi.
5. http://www.homeoint.org/cazalent/tyler/hayfever.htm
6. H C Allen; 2004; *Allen's Keynotes* - Rearranged and Classified, Reprint Ed.; B Jain Publishers, New Delhi.
7. William Boericke; 2003; *Homoeopathic Materia Medica and Repertory*, Reprint Ed.; B Jaion Publishers, New Delhi
8. http://www.homeopathic.com/articles/using_h/allergies_resp.php

CHAPTER 21

Homeopathic Management of Non-allergic Rhinitis - A Case Analysis

Several patients who visit our free clinics run by **Dr Rangachari** in Singapore, have been treated for symptoms of non-allergic rhinitis. When they came for consultation, they were heavily dependent on anti-histamines to carry on their normal daily work. There was no known allergic cause for the symptoms. They have shown good progress after homeopathic treatment and their consumption of anti-histamines has reduced dramatically.

His complete case analysis of a patient who stopped taking antitistomines after taking homeopathic treatment, is presented below.

DETAILS OF CASE

Name : Mr. X.

Age : 28

Nationality : Indian

Status : Married

Occupation : Technician

Work Environment : He works in an air conditioned environment which he finds very chilly.

Chief Complaint : Sneezing; running nose; eyes red and watering, every day
- Sneezing episodes every day after waking up in the morning
- Sneezes about 50 times or more throughout the day - feels it is due to the strong air conditioning in the office. Finds it difficult to work because of sneezing
- Sometimes, itching inside the nose is followed by sneezing.
- Sneezing more in the day and much less at night; able to sleep quite well
- Copious watery discharge from the nose and the handkerchief becomes wet
- Sometimes nose becomes blocked
- Often the eyes become red accompanied by burning and lachrymation
- After too much sneezing, patient has headche and body pain
- Worse in the air conditioned environment. Better outdoors
- Had this problem since 3 years (after coming to Singapore). Sneezing is much less when he goes to india
- He had to take anti-histamines every day and wants to stop their usage

Other Complaints
- Headache because of sneezing
- Head feels heavy; sensation like water moving in the head from side to when head is moved
- Body pain, especially joints, legs and hands
- Feverish feeling, but no fever

Mentals : Anxiety due to family responsibilities; feeling home-sickness.

Homeopathic Management of Non-allergic Rhinitis - A Case Analysis

Past History : Tendency to take cold easily.

Family History : Mother has asthma, hypertension and diabetes. Grandmother and elder brother have asthma. Elder brother also takes cold easily and has eosonophilia. Father has diabetes.

Physical Appearance and Examination
- **Appearance :** Slightly dark complexioned, medium stature, slender build
- **Examination :** Eyes slightly red, on first visit; snuffles now and then

First Prescription (Before Repertorigation)

Based on acute symptoms, the patient was prescribed *Sabadilla* 30C and was asked to return after a week.

CASE ANALYSIS

Chief Complaint : Chronic and recurrent rhinitis. Now persistent, causing difficulties at work and home.

Miasmatic Analysis
- **Past History :** Patient is prone to catch cold - suggests a tubercular background
- **Family History :** Mother, grandmother and elder brother have asthma; both mother and father have diabetes - suggests sycotic family background
- Current tendency for persistent rhinitis symptoms indicates that the active miasm may be psoric or tubercular.

ANALYSIS AND CLASSIFICATION OF SYMPTOMS
Mental Generals

1. *Anxiety* due to family responsibilities.
2. Home-sick feelings.
3. Slight resentment due to family disputes.
4. Likes and feels better in open space / open air.

Physical Generals
1. Slender build of medium height.
2. Thirst, appetite, stools, sleep are normal.
3. Likes salty food, but avoids it for health reasons.
4. Thermal status - no preference for cold or warm weather.
5. Sweats more on back and chest.
6. Feverish feeling, but no fever.

Particulars

Eyes
- Quite often, the eyes become red (at least once a day).
- *Eyes watering and irritated,* even when not sneezing.
- Burning sensation in the eyes.
- Tears when coughing or sneezing.

Nose
- Sneezing episodes every day after waking up in the morning
- Sneezes about 50 times or more, throughout the day - feels it is due to the strong air conditioning in the office
- Sometimes, itching inside the nose is followed by sneezing
- Sneezing more in the day and much less at night; able to sleep quite well
- Copious watery discharge from the nose making the handkerchief wet
- Nose blocked; sometimes, both nostrils are blocked

Head
- *Headache on sides* because of too much sneezing
- Head feels heavy

- Sensation like water moving in the head from side to side when head is moved

Extremities
- Joint pain in legs and hands

Modalities
- > *In air conditioned environment;* by taking cold fruits from the refrigerator
- > In open spaces; in the absence of air conditioning

EVALUATION OF SYMPTOMS (GRADING/CHOOSING SYMPTOMS FOR REPERTORIZATION)

Since the mental or physical generals are not very pronounced, only the particulars are taken for repertorization. Symptoms in *italics* are converted to rubrics and repertorised.

Particulars

Eyes
- *Red*
- *Lachrymation*
- *Tears when coughing or sneezing*
- *Burning sensation*

Nose
- *Sneezing episodes* on waking up and throughout the day
- *Itching inside the nose*
- *Copious watery discharge from the nose*
- *Nose blocked quite often;* sometimes both are nostrils
- Sneezing more in the day and less at night

Head
- *Head feels heavy;* pain in the sides

- Sensation like water moving in the head from side to side when head is moved

Modalities
- > In air conditioned environment, by taking cold fruits from the refrigerator
- > In open spaces; in the absence of air conditioning

REPERTORIZATION

Using Kent's Repertory

Conversion of Chosen Symptoms to Rubrics

Chosen symptoms	No.	Rubrics from Kent's Reoestosy	Page No.
Redness of eyes	1	Eye, redness, lids, edges of	265
Lachrymation	2	Eye, lachrymation	245
Tears with coughing	3	Eye, lachrymationm, cough, with	245
Frequent bouth of sneezing	4	Nose, sneezing, paroxysmal	351
Nose blocked	5	Nose, obstruction	340
Watery discharge	6	Nose, discharge, copious	330
Itching inside the nose	7	Nose, itching, inside	339
Heaviness in head	8	Head, heaviness, sides	127
Aggravated by air conditioned room	9	Generalities, cold, air agg.	1348

Results of Repertorization - Group of Remedies to be Considered

Remedy	Marks/No. of Symptoms Covered
Arsenicum	16/6
Euphrasia	11/5
Natrium mur.	19/8
Nux vom.	14/7
Sabadilla	17/9
Pulsatilla	15/6
Sulphur	18/7

Second Prescription - Remedies Chosen on Second Visit

For Miasmatic treatment - *Sulphur* 200C / one dose

For Acute Symptoms - The remedy chosen - *Natrium mur.* 30C alternating with *Sabadilla* 30C for 10 days.

JUSTIFICATION OF CHOICE OF REMEDY

- According to the above repertorisation, the remedy of choice can be Sabadilla, Natrium mur. and Sulphur
- Natrium mur. has the maximum marks, but covers, 8 symptoms whereas Sabadilla has 17 marks and covers all the nine symptoms. Both remedies cover the impotant nose and eye symptoms quite well since the patient had earlier responded well to Sabadilla, it was decided to continue Sabadilla, but alternate it with Natrium mur.
- The next choice is Sulphur which gets 18 marks and covers 7 symptoms. Sulphur is a very good anti-psoric and deep acting remedy, whereas Sabadilla is only a short acting remedy. Hence, one dose of Sulphur 200 was prescribed, as the miasmatic remedy.
- Although, *Arsenicum* has good marks, it covers only six symptoms
- The more important nasal symptoms are not fully covered by *Pulsatilla* (15 marks) or *Euphrasia* (11 marks)
- Natrium mur., which has covered most of the symptoms so well, is also kept in mind as a possible *constitutional remedy* for future treatment.

POTENCY AND DOSAGE PRESCRIBED

First Visit (Before Repertorisation)

Sabadilla 30C - TDS daily.

Second Visit (After Repertorization)

After two weeks, the condition improved and sneezing was down by 70 percent. Second prescription after repertorization Sulphur 200 - one dose *Natrium mur.* 30C twice in the morning and *Sabadilla* 30C twice in the evening, for 10 days.

Third Visit

After two weeks. As the sneezing became less and less, dosage was reduced gradually and then medication was stopped.

Fourth Visit

After one month, the symptoms returned, but with less intensity.

Psorinum 1M - one dose as intercurrent.

Natsium mur. 30C in the morning and Sabadilla 30C in the evening, as and when required.

COMPLEMENTARY REMEDIES

In addition to homeopathic medicine, the following were prescribed during the first visit:

- Bach flower - Rescue Remedy (for mental well being), TDS daily.

LIFE STYLE ADVICE

Patient was advised as follows:
- Stop drinking cold beverages or cold water from the refrigerator
- Try steam inhalation often a relieve blockage of nose
- Try yoga exercises such as *Jala neti* and breathing exercises
- Wear woolens in the air conditioned environment

MIASMATIC AND CONSTITUTIONAL TREATMENT

- The active miasm is Psora as indicated by the present symptoms. The patient has responded well to Sulphur, Natrium mur. and Psorium, all of which are excellent anti-psorics.
- The patient has a sycotic background with a family history of diabetes and asthma. He also has a tendency to catch cold often. Hence, the future treatment under consideration is one or two doses of *Tuberculinum* 200C (or 1M) alternating with *Sulphur* 200C (or 1M).
- This is be followed by a long-term constitutional treatment (Probably with *Natrium mur.*). Since this is a chronic case of rhinitis, constitutional treatment would be beneficial (after the mental picture becomes more clear).

MANAGEMENT AND PROGNOSIS

To summarise, the patient has a history of paroxysmal sneezing since 3 year without any relief. The active miasm is psoric and he responded very well to Natrium mur. 30C, Sabadilla 30C, Sulphur 200C. When the sneezing cleared up, and the patient was entirely free of symptoms for more than a month.

When the symptoms returned with lesser intensity, he was prescribed one dose of Psorinum 1M as intercurrent and Natrium mur. 30C alternating with Sabadilla 30C as before. *He* has not taken antihistamines for more than 3 months now and is happy with the homeopathic treatment.

Prognosis seem to be good since his dependency on antihistamines has ceased and it is likely that he will be relived of the recurring symptoms of rhinitis after completing the miasmatic as well as the constitutional treatment.

Bibliography

1. James Tyler Kent; 2004; *Repertory of the Homeopathic Materia Medica,* Reprint Ed.; B. Jain Publishers, New Delhi.
2. William Boericke; *Homeopathic Materia Medica and Repertory,* Reprint Ed.; B Jain Publishers, New Delhi.
3. S K Banerjea; 2003; *Miasmatic Diagnosis,* Reprint Ed.; B Janin Publishers, New Delhi.

CHAPTER 22

Some Interesting Case Studies In Brief

CASE I

Name : Mrs Y

Age : 44 years

Nationality : Indian

Sex : Female

Marital status : Married

Occupation : Housemaid

Chief Complaint : Sneezing; running nose; eyes red and watering, on most of the days.

The patient came for the first time in 2004 with severe rhinitis. Incessant sneezing early in the morning, watery eyes, blocked nose at night, headaches. Not particularly allergic to dust or spices in the kitchen. Cause of sneezing not known.

She was a housemaid and so all the usual problems of being away from home were expected. Instead, she was happy to be away from home due to family problems and marital problems. She was short tempered, would be rude to her employer sometimes and disliked consolation.

She was reluctant to try homeopathy but had no choice as her employer insisted that she should try it as conventional medicines were giving her no relief.

Medication

She was given *Natrium mur.* 200C, to take everyday for a week and later to slowly reduce to one dose. She was also given Biochemic salts and Rescue Remedy.

The employer reported that although there was some improvement, the maid could not be monitored to take her medication as she later was disinclined for treatment.

The maid came on and off over a period of one year without much improvement and one wondered whether she was taking the medication at all.

The breakthrough came in late 2005, when the maid came back on her own to give homeopathy an honest try. A detailed case taking was once again done.

She was a fastidious patient, given to cleaning, very chilly, allergic to dust, felt better with warm drinks.

Psorinum 200 was given as an intercurrent remedy. Two weeks later the employer called to say that there was remarkable improvement in the maid's condition.

After nearly 3 months, the maid came back as her symptoms were returning but in a milder form. *Arsericum alb* 200C and *Sabadilla* 30C have helped her and there is a steady improvement in the condition. She was prescribed *Tuberculinum* 1M in August 2006 and is under observation.

CASE II

Name : Master Z

Age : 9 years

Sex : Male

Patient - 9-year old male child.

Chief Complaint : Recurrent attacks of sneezing and cold since 7 years, leading to fever on many occasions.

Symptoms :
- Rhinitis. Chilly patient.
- Stubborn; sensitive. Aversion to curd; craving for chocolates
- Perspiration increased on head < night
- Active child, lean and thin build

Tubercular miasm is to be considered because of recurrence and step-by-step developement of the disease. It started with sneezing and led to discharge from the nose and later produced cough and fever.

Treatment

The diagnosis that the case was rhinitis (allergic?) with a tubercular background. The child was prescribed *Natrium phos.* (an unusual prescription for rhinitis), which totally relieved him within three months.

CASE III

Name : Mrs. W

Age : 28 years

Sex : Female

Marital Status : Married

Occupation : Housewife

Chief Complaint : Sneezing; running nose; coryza, for the last 8 years.

Totality Derived :
- Attack always started with irritation in nose, followed by continuous sneezing, runny nose with clear watery mucus discharge, lachrymation
- Great catarrhal headache at the forehead
- Profuse lachrymation, burning of eyes > in open air
- Attack by touch of water of damp air; when entering from open air to warm room or from warm room to cold air
- > When walding continously in open air; cut < morning and evening; > in moderate temperature; > by covering or wrapping head with warm cloth; < when working in kitchen, hoste
- Great pain at the root of nose and eyebrows, sometimes stuffy and lumpy feeling at the root of nose.
- Pain in feet, ankles when working in water; gets tired easily; pain in joints.

Treatment

Allium cepa 30, FP 6X, CP 3X, NM 3X, Sil. 12X alternating with above medicine for 10 days.

Follow ups
- After 10 days, one dose of *Bacillinum* 200 days and later *Allium cepa* was repeated one in 20 days
- Then *Silicea* 1M two doses after every three weeks
- The patient did not complain again

CASE IV

An interesting case of rhinitis along with urticaria.

Name : Mrs. Y

Age : 40 years

Sex : Female

Chief Complaint : Sneezing; running nose; urticaria.

Symptoms :

- Urticaria since 6 years aggravated by anxiety and thinking. She had to take anti-allergic drugs frequently for the same
- *Sneezing with running nose, aggravated in morning*
- Pain in small joints of hands, ameliorated by warmth and pressure
- Recurrent sore throats with feverish sensation, accompanied by weakness and bitter taste in mouth
- Past medical history: Rheumatic fever
- Personality ; She was basically an introvert lady with a very scientific and active mind. She was a logical thinker. She would go into depth of each subject she studied. She was a topper throughout her academic carrer. She was a perfectionist. She had a complaint of claustrophobia; fear that she will be suffocated. She was very time bound, always anxious about time. She couldn't and any disorder. She couldn't tolerate cold weather.

Treatment :

After a detailed anaysis of her case she was prescribed a dose of *Arsenicum alb.* 1M and she was called after 1 week of her follow up.

Follow ups :

Follow up after 1 week – She complained of increased sneezing and nasal discharge.

In her third visit after 15 days her urticaria and her joint pains were much better and with each subsequent visit her condition got better with no complaints left.

CASE V

Name : Mr R.
Sex : Male
Patient - Male
Chief Complaint - Sneezing, cold (+3), lachrymation and watery nasal discharge since the last 6 months.

Totality Derived -
- The sneezing starts suddenly and it is aggravated after bathing (+3), cold drinks, change of weather, dust mites
- If he takes warm tea he feels relieved for sometime
- During this episode he feels cold +3. He has an aversion to fanning
- He feels thirsty and takes about one glass of water at a time
- Currently he is working in his father's manufacturing unit of liquid fertilizers
- He has a marked fear of darkness and ghosts

Treatment
1. *Arsencium.* 30, 3 powders at night.
2. S. L 30, TDS, for 7 days

Follow ups -

After one week : Feeling better. Watery discharge from nose better

O/e Throat congested (+3). Same treatment condinued for another week.

Third week : Retrosternal burning - *Nux vomica* 30 powder was given, rest was S. L. for 7 days.

On subsequent visits, patient was better; No throat congestion. He was put on placebo.

The patient called after 6 months just to inform that he has been well all these days.

CHAPTER **23**

Supplementary Therapies - Biochemic Salts and Bach Flower Remedies

"The patient is the most important factor in his healing".

- Dr. Hahnemann

ROLE OF SUPPLEMENTARY THERAPIES

Homeopathic treatment can be effectively supplemented by Biochemics and Bach flower remedies[1]. While biochemic salts are capable of functioning at a physiological level, the Bach flower remedies provide excellent support by correcting the emotional and mental imbalances in the patient.

I. Biochemic Therapeutics

Biochemic salts are also known as the *Tissue salts*. Discovered by **Dr. Schussler** in 1873, this system of medicine is based on the theory that *disease is caused by the insufficiency of certain salts in the tissues/cells of the body and that disease can be cured by the supply of the appropriate salt(s)*. Thus the physiological basis of *Biochemic therapeutics* is the requirement of certain inorganic constituents and their appropriate distribution to ensure the proper functioning and vitality of the organs. These salts remain after combustion of the tissues and tissues and from the ashes.

Schussler was *himself a homeopath* and he identified *12 basic salts* as biochemic remedies. These are:

1. Calcarea fluorica (Calcium fluoride)
2. Calcarea phosphoricum (Calcium phosphate)
3. Calcarea sulphuricum (calcium sulphate)
4. Ferrum phosphoricum (Iron phosphate)
5. Kalium muriaticum (Potassium chloride)
6. Kalium phosphoricum (Potassium phosphate)
7. Kalium sulphuricum (Potassium sulphate)
8. Magnesium phosphoricum (Magnesium phosphate)
9. Natrium sulphuricum (Glauber's salt - Sodium sulphate)
10. Natrium phosphoricum (Sodium phosphate)
11. Silicea (Silica)

These inorganic constituents are absolutely essential for maintaining the integrity of structure and functional activity of the organs and tissues in the body. According to Schussler's theory, any distubance in the molecular motion of these salts in living tissues, caused by a deficiency in the requisite amount, constitutes disease. Administering the same mineral salts is small quantities can rectify this and re-establish the required equilibrium. Analysis has shown that the twelve tissue salts are also constituents of many well know homeopathic remedies of the vegetable kingdom.

Prescription

These salts are *triturated,* but generally prescribed in a very low potency, such as $3x$, $6x$, $12x$, etc. It is advisable to start the medicine with low potency ($3x$) and proceed to higher potencies ($6x$, $12x$, $30x$, etc) in case there is no improvement. The selected remedy, dissolved in water, is very effective as well. For severe problems, higher potencies may be used to start the treatment. Dosage is three times a day (4-6 pills at a time) generally. In acute problems, the medicine may be taken every 15 minutes or half-an-hour. If there is no improvement even after 6-7 doses, the prescription can be changed.

Biochemic Salts for Nose Symptoms in Rhinitis

Biochemic salts provide *useful supportive therapy*, especially in the children. Most to the salts have well defined nasal symptoms, the most remarkable among them being *Natrium mur.* They are useful when a mild medication is required.

Boericke and Dewey have listed the following symptoms under therapeutic applications:

Natrium muriaticum
- Much sneezing, worse on undressing at night and in morning
- Catarrhs and colds with watery, transparent, frothy discharge
- Running cold, worse by going into the cold and by exertion
- Loss of sense of smell
- Posterior nares dry
- Frontal sinus inflammation
- Epistaxis from stooping and cough
- Fever

Ferrum phosphoricum
Congestion of nasal mucus membranes, incipient colds, smarting in nasal passages (especially the right), worse on inspiration, predisposition to take cold, feverish conditions.

Calcarea phosphoricum
Sneezing and sore nostrils, chronic catarrhal conditions,

nasal polyps, point of nose icy cold, albuminous discharge fluent in cold room, stopped in warm air and outdoors, pressure at the root of nose with frontal headache.

Calcarea fluorica
Stuffy cold and ineffectual desire to sneeze.

Natrium sulphuricum
Catarrhs of mucous membranes in general is characterized by a tendency to profuse secretion of greenish mucus stuffing up of nose.

Kalium phosphoricum
Sneezes from the slightest exposure, thick mucus hawked from posterior nares.

Kalium sulphuricum
Loss of smell, nose obstructed, yellowish discharge.

Magnesium phosphoricum
Alternate dry and loose coryza, *gushing flow from nostrils.*

Natrium phosphoricum
Pricking in the nares, itching of nose, tension over root of nose, catarrh with thick discharge.

Silicea
Sneezing, tip of nose red, itching of nostrils, painful, chronic dryness of nose, acrid, corroding discharge, intolerable itching of tip of nose.

Kalium muriaticum
Thick white discharge, stuffy cold.

II. Bach Flower Remedies
Dr. Edward Bach (1889-1936) believed that there is an

intimate co-relation between physical ailments and the mental state of the patient. In the 1930s, he devised a new method of treatment which makes use of 38 remedies to cover the various negative states of mind that mankind suffers from.

Dr. Bach classified people under seven major emotional groups such as fear, uncertainty, loneliness, etc. Using his knowledge of homeopathy, he then formulated 38 unique flower-based remedies to treat each emotional state, as indicated below.

Seven Major Emotional Groups

1. Fear
- Terror - **Rock rose**
- Fear of unknown things - **Mimulus**
- Fear of mind giving way - **Cherry plum**
- Fears and worries of unknown origin - **Aspen**
- Fear or over-concern for others - **Red chestnut**

2. Loneliness
- Proud, aloof - **Water Violet**
- Impatience - **Impatiens**
- Self-centredness, self concern - **Heather**

3. Insufficient Interest in Present Circumstances
- Dreaminess, lock of interest in present - **Clematis**
- Lives in the past - **Honeysuckle**
- Resignation, apathy - **Wild rose**
- Lack of energy - **Olive**
- Unwanted thoughts, mental arguments - **White chestnut**
- Deep gloom with no origin - **Mustard**
- Failure to learn from past mistakes - **Chestnut bud**

4. Despondency or Despair

- Lack of confidence - **Larch**
- Self-reproach, guilt - **Pine**
- Overwhelmed by responsibility - **Elm**
- Extreme mental anguis - **Sweet chestnut**
- After-effects of shock - **Star of Bethlehem**
- Resentment - **Willow**
- Exhausted but struggles on - **Oak**
- Self-hatred, sense of uncleanliness - **Crab apple**

5. Uncertainty
- Seeks advice and confirmation from others - **Cerato**
- Indecision - **Scleranthus**
- Discouragement, despondency - **Gentian**
- Hopelessness and dispair - **Gorse**
- "Monday morning" feeling - **Hornbeam**
- Uncertainty as to the correct path in life - **Wild oat**

6. Over Sensitivity to Influences and Ideas
- Mental torment behind a brave face - **Agrimony**
- Weak-willed and subservient - **Centaury**
- Protection from change and outside influences - **Walnut**
- Hatred, envy, jealousy - **Holly**

7. Over-care for the Welfare of Others
- Selfishly possessive - **Chicory**
- Over-enthusiasm - **Vervain**
- Dominating, inflexible - **Vine**
- Intolerance - **Beech**
- Self-repression, self-denial - **Rock Water**

Rescue Remedy

In addition to these, another popular flower remedy is the well-know *Rescue Remedy*, which is a unique combination of five

Bach flower remedies:

Rock rose - for terror, *Impatiens* - for impatience, *Clematis* - for dreaminess; lack of interest in the present, *Star of Bethlehem* - for the after-effects of shock, *Cherry plum* - for fear of the mind giving way.

For Rhinitis Patients

Rescue remedy and other individual flower remedies offer good support during homeopathic treatment of rhinitis patients. For instance, several patients who indicated that they suffer from repetitive thought patterns have been prescribed *White chestnut* along with *Rescue remedy*.

Other individual remedies are also prescribed according to the emotional state of the patient as indicated in the above scheme.

REFERENCES

1. http://www.homeoint.org/site/deepak/biochemic/htm#bio
2. W Boericke and W A Dewey, *The Twelve Tissue Remedies of Schussler*, Reprint Ed.; B. Jain Publishers, New Delhi
3. R L Gupta; 2000; *Unique Combinations with Clinical Cases in Homeopathy and Biochemic*, Reprint Ed.; B Jain Publishers, New Delhi
4. http://homeoint.org/site/ahmad/schuessler.htm
5. http://homeoint.org/site/ahmad/biochemic.htm
6. http://www.hpathy.com/tissuesalts/biochemic-theory.asp
7. http://www.bachcentre.com/centre/remedies.htm
8. http://www.internethealthlibrary.com/Therapies/BachFlowerRemedies.htm

CHAPTER **24**

Alternative Methods: A Holistic Approach

WHAT IS AN ALTERNATIVE THERAPY?

It is better to define alternative therapies in terms of them having non-scientific explanations. In so far as a therapy does have a biological explanation, it should be regarded as simply part of orthodox medicine. The crucial difference between orthodox and alternative therapies is therefore that alternative medical systems have non-scientific explanations based on spiritual, mystical, legendary or otherwise intuitively-appealing insights.

This difference between orthodox and alternative medicine can be illustrated with an example. In orthodox medicine, the illness of 'hypertension' or high blood pressure is explained in terms of a mass of inter-linked biological knowledge concerning the structure and function of the human body including heart and arteries and the functional relationship between blood pressure and diseases such as stroke. Drug treatment of hypertension is based on a detailed scientific understanding of how the heart and arteries are regulated by the nervous system, and how this can be modified using drugs. The fact that orthodox therapies are embedded in standard biological science is what makes them scientifically testable.

By contrast, acupuncture is based around the existence of meridians, which are structures described in historic medical and religious literature but not detectable using scientific equipment. In homoeopathy, the mechanism of action is based on a 'magical' form of reasoning – the 'law of similars', or like-cures-like - which has no basis in modern therapeutics. Another homoeopathic principle, that of increasing potency of a medicine with increasing dilution (so long as dilution is done in a particular way called succussion) is in contradiction with modern chemistry. And in chiropractic medicine, the presumed spinal vertebral subluxations which are supposed to cause disease are not visible using imaging technologies such as X-rays or MRI scans. Yet acupuncture, homoeopathy and chiropractic are among the most professionalized of alternative therapies – the explanatory theories for crystal healing or aromatherapy are even more imaginative and less scientific. This means that Alternative medical systems are unconstrained by existing scientific knowledge even where they do not actually contradict current science.

WHY ALTERNATIVE METHODS?

Several new over-the-counter (OTC) drugs promise fast relief of rhinitis symptoms without drowsiness.

> *"Take this wonder pill, they say,*
> *and be smiling night and day!"*

However, patients afflicted with allergic or non-allergic know that it is not that simple. Millions of people who suffer from nasal symptoms as in rhinitis are heavily dependent on anti-histamines and anti-inflammatory drugs. Several patients experience some sort of side effects because of these medications and are reluctant to start steroid treatment. These patients are often very earnest in seeking some alternative treatment that can provide long-term relief.

A wide range of simple and convenient methods of

alternative treatment or management are available for such long-suffering patients of persistent rhinitis. These methods offer a *holistic approach* to the problem and are worth trying it out in the long run. These include:

- Nasal irrigation with saline solution
- Non-prescription nasal sprays
- Yoga - Jala neti exercise
- Yoga - Breathing exercises (such as Pranayama) and asanas
- Naturopathy combined with yoga
- Ayurveda
- TCM - Traditionl Chinese Medicine
- Acupuncture
- Tai chi

CHAPTER **25**

Nasal Wash and Nasal Sprays

a. Nasal Irrigation with Saline Solution

Nose and sinuses may be washed with salt water in this simple and convenient procedure. Nasal irrigation utilizing a buffered hypertonic saline solution helps to *reduce swollen and congested nasal and sinus tissues.* In addition, it washes out thickened nasal secretions, irritants (smog, pollens, etc.), bacteria, and crusts from the nose and sinuses. Non-prescription nasal sprays (Ocean spray, Ayr, nasal) can be used frequently, and are very convenient.

Procedure

Nasal irrigation can be done several times a day, and is frequently performed with a syringe or a Water Pik device (the attachment is purchased separately). The irrigating solution can be made by adding 2-3 heaped teaspoons of salt to one pint of water. It is best to use Marten Coarse Kosher Salt or Springfield plain salt because table salt may have unwanted additives. To this solution, add 1 teaspoon of baking soda. Store at room temperature and always mix the solution before use.

If the solution stings, use less salt. In the beginning, or for children, it is best to start with a weaker salt mixture. Initially, it is not unusual, to have a mild burning sensation irrigation. While irrigating the nose, it is best to stand over the sink and irrigate each side of the nose. Aim the stream toward the back of head, not at the top of head. For young children, the salt water can be put into a small spray container which can be squirted several times into each nostril.

b. Non-prescription Nasal Sprays

Spraying with Capsaicin (From Capsicum Pepper)

Capsaicin is a phenolic chemical contained within the oil of the Capsicum pepper. Capsaicin is initially very irritating to its targeted area. However, the area becomes desensitized to the irritation after repeated use. The nerve responsible for rhinorrhea, sneezing and congestion become desensitized when Capsaicin is applied to the nasal mucosa. Therefore, symptoms are halted. Capsaicin is adviced to patients presenting with congestion, rhinorrhea, sneezing, or a combination of these symptoms. Clinical studies have revealed a 60% reduction in nasal airway resistance.

Silver Nitrate (For Topical Use)

Although, Silver Nitrate is not widely implemented in clinical practice, topically applied silver nitrate is believed to *regulate nasal mucous membranes to stimuli* through a local astringent action of coagulated albumin. Patients presenting with rhinorrhea, sneezing and congestion are most likely to benefit from silver nitrate.

CHAPTER 26

Yoga Therapy

HISTORY OF YOGA THERAPY

Yoga has been used in traditional Indian medicine for thousands of years. However, Yoga therapy in its present form is a new discipline, created by the marriage of traditional Yoga with modern medicine. Swami Kuvalyananda pioneered Yoga therapy in the early 1920s, applying the methods of modern medical science to study the physiological effects and therapeutic application of Yoga and, in the following decades, his practices spread to the rest of India & World.

YOGA THERAPY APPLICATION

Yoga comprises a wide range of mind/body practices, ranging from postural and breathing exercises to deep relaxation and meditation. Yoga therapy tailors these to the health needs of individuals. It promotes all round total health, as well as helping particular medical conditions. Yoga offers an excellent training program for the purpose of maintaining one's health. Regular practice of Yoga, for minimum 30 to 45 minutes daily, helps not only in developing a physical fitness but also, in preventing the occurrence of many such ailments which invariably result from hectic pace of modern life style.

Yogic practices are very effective in the treatment if various functional and Psycho-physiological disorders. When Yogic practices are used either as a complimentary or as in some cases, even as a substitute to the conventional treatment, it definitely leads to a long term relief and possible permanent cure.

Our object is to develop a clear and rationale understanding of various Yogic techniques, on educating the individual in identifying the unhealthy elements in their day to day living which contribute in their problem and holding them in correcting the factors.

YOGA FOR RHINITIS

This may be discussed under two heads:
 (a) Jala neti exercise
 (b) Breathing exercises & asanas

a. Yog - Jala Neti Exercise

For patients plagued with problems of rhinitis and sinusitis for years, the *jal neti* exercise is a boon.

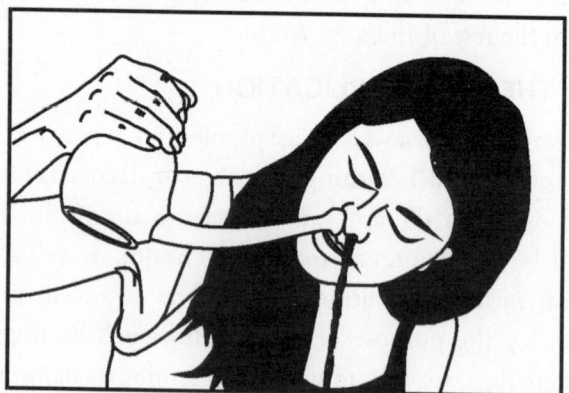

Fig. 1.1 – Jal Neti

Neti - Nasal cleansing as in Hatha Yoga

One of the simplest yet powerful method, the ancient technique of *jal neti* can be a useful yogic tool to ward off the nasal symptoms *and keep the nasal passages clear at all time.* Neti works wonders *for all kinds of nasal complaints like sinusitis, chronic rhinitis, allergies, and in several cases for asthma.* (Neti also helps in relieving headaches and facilitates in maintaining youthfulness. It has a remarkable effect upper over the respiratory tract infections).

Kriyas form the mainstay in the yogic management of nasal symptoms. Neti is actually one of the six classical kriyas (cleansing practices) mentioned in the *Hatha Yoga Pradipika and the Gheranda Samhita,* although the technique mentioned by both texts is actually *Sutra neti* (done with a cotton thread or a catheter) rather gentler technique of *Jala neti* (sometimes called Saline Nasal Irrigation), in which warm salt water is used. According to both texts, Neti "cleanses the skull, induces clairvoyance and removes diseases that are above the shoulders". It also greatly enchances olfactory sensitivity and is an important therapeutic concept in the treatment of upper respiratory tract ailments. It supports and reactivates the nasal mucosa cleansing mechanisms.

The Methodology

Jal neti helps in controlling the over-reactive lining of the nose. When Jal neti is done voluntarily, it provides training to the nose to tolerate the irritant (the saline water), and in this process, nose learns to tolerate other irritants also such as dust or pollen or cold air. Once learnt, the practice can be done in about 3 minutes and is easily integrated into a daily routine of body cleansing such as showering or cleaning of the teeth.

1. First, the *Neti* pot is filled with water at the right temperature and degree of salinity.

   Some points to remember are:
   - Good quality sea salt should be used. Salt is often mixed with anticaking agents which gives it an unpleasant taste (or smell). Make sure you use good quality, pure sea salt.

- *It is very important that the right amount of salt is put in the water.* The water should taste salty, but not overty. Too little or too much salt is extremely uncomfortable and possibly even dangerous (it can sometimes cause nose bleed)
- As a rough guideline, 1 table spoon for one litre of water is sufficient.
- The water temperature has to be comfortable (it should be at body temperature, or a little cooler).

2. Bend forward and then tilt head head from side to side.
3. The spout of the pot is inserted into one nostril. The position of the head and pot are adjusted to allow the water to flow out of the other nostril.
4. Relax, breathe through the mouth and pour gently the salted water through the upper nostril. *The water will flow around the septum and out through the other nostril.*
5. Do not inhale as you pour the water through come the nose.
6. Pour half the water through one nostril, then blow your nose vigorously before tilting the head the other way and repeating the operation for the other nostril.
7. Once this is finished, it is important to thoroughly dry the nasal passages with a few rounds of *Kapalabhati* (rapid breathing with forced abdominal exhalation).

The operation only takes a couple of minutes is not as uncomfortable as one might imagine at first, and its benefits are such that it is well worth including *Jala neti* in the daily routine.

[For those who are nervous about getting it right, EMCUR, a German company, manufactures a very user-friendly system which includes a nasal douche and pre-packed salt portions. A bit more expensive than an ordinary neti pot, but totally safe!]

b. Yoga - Breathing Exercises and Asanas

According to Yoga, nasal reactions to irritants are considered a manifestation of a minor imbalance in prana and hence very quick results can be seen in people who practice an integrated approach of Yoga therapy. The ancient art of yoga affect several *techniques of asanas such as Padangusthasana* to overcome nasal allergies caused by reactions to various external stimuli. Regular practice of breathing exercises and asanas help to overcome nasal symptoms.

Recommended exercises are:
- Tiger breathing, rabbit, sasankasana breathing
- Loosening exercises (jogging, twisting)
- Yogasanas
- Suryanamaskara (12 postures in standing, sittting, prone and supine positions) and pranayama.
- Meditation along with a lifestyle change through jnana, karma and bhakti yoga

TIGER BREATHING
Benefits
Tiger pose warms and stretches the back muscles and spine. Tiger pose strengthens the core body and stimulates the nervous, lymphatic and reproductive systems.

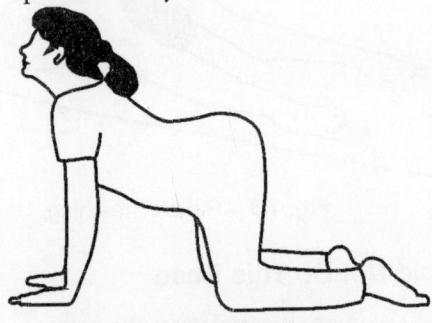

Fig. 1.2 – Tiger Breathing

Steps

1. From table position, inhale the right knee to the forehead, rounding the spine
2. Exhale reach the right foot up towards the ceiling, arching the spine and looking up at the ceiling.
3. Inhale the forehead to knee and exhale the foot up 4-8 times, then repeat on the left side.
4. To release: exhale the knee back down to the floor into table position.
5. Place a folded blanket under the knees to protect them from pressure and stress.

CONTRAINDICATION

Recent or chronic injury to the back, hips, or knees

RABBIT BREATHING

This is a wonderful pose for releasing the neck, shoulders and lower back! It stretches the entire neck, including up to where the neck joins the skull. It's one of the few yoga poses that loosens under the shoulder blades. It releases tension in the trapezius muscles. It stretches out the lower back. Great for headaches!

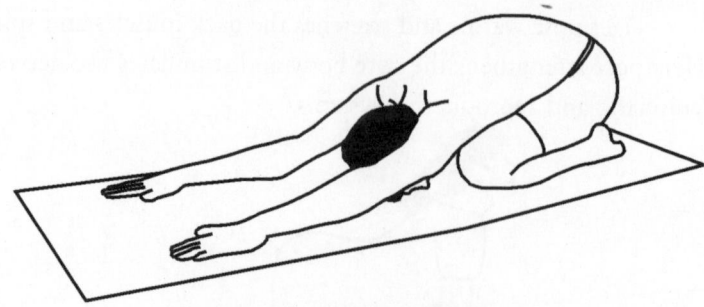

Fig. 1.3 – Rabbit Breathing

Who Should Not Do This Pose

Pregnant women. It compresses the belly too much. However,

you'll hardly need the warning, since there's not much chance you'll want to do it after the fourth month!

Start - from Child Pose, like this:

Sitting on your knees:
- Elongate your spine.
- Stretch your body forward over your legs.
- Curl you head between your knees.
- Rest the top of your head or your forehead on the floor.
- Arms rest by your sides, hands by your feet.
- Allow your shoulders to drop toward the floor and relax.
- Let the weight in your body drop downward.
- In this opening position you might feel a gentle stretch in your lower back and shoulders.

Key Stretching your body forward along your legs before you curl under is a key part of getting the most out of the Rabbit.

Tip You'll get the best stretch the more your head is curled under and the more your nose is tucked between your knees.

Next

Hold onto your heels. Have all your fingers and your thumbs on the outside of the heels.

Bring your hips upward.

If your shoulders and lower back allow it, you continue to bring your hips upward until your arms are straight.

To increase the stretch, keep trying to bring your hips more upward.

You'll feel some of your weight rolling onto the top of your head. If that is uncomfortable for you, you can straighten your head a little.

Tip If you allow your head to rotate, curling it more under your body, you can increase the stretch in your neck and lower back. If you get an extreme stretch and want even more, you can tuck your head into your knees farther.

Modifications

Release by reversing your movements, letting your hips down and returning your arms to your sides.

If you cannot reach your feet, use a yoga strap or belt. This is one of the few poses where I freely recommend using props. There are few ways to modify this pose without one.

If you have trouble sitting in the opening Child Pose without your neck or shoulders or thighs resisting, try using a firm cushion or a rolled up yoga mat to support your head.

Breathing

Sitting on your knees, **breathe in & out** as you settle into place

Breathing in, elongate your spine.

Breathing out, stretch your body forward along your knees, curling your head under. Breathe in and out as you settle into place.

Breathe in as you go into the Rabbit

Hold the pose as you breathe in and out.

While You Hold the Pose

Breathing in, see if you can increase the stretch by coaxing your hips up farther.

Breathing out, feel the weight in your shoulders and legs sinking and relaxing, without losing any of the stretch.

Release the pose as you breathe out.

Primary Suryanamaskara

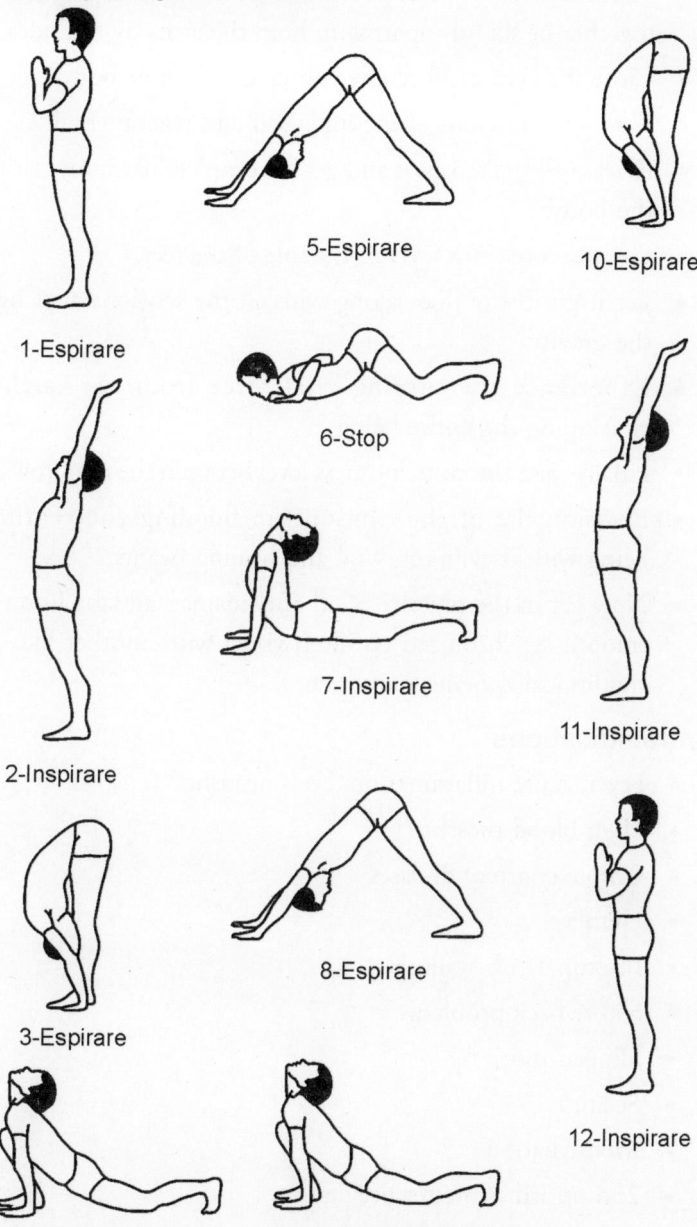

Fig. 1.4 – Primary Suryanamaskara

- Stand up in relaxed posture, either holding the feet together or slightly apart with both the arms by the sides.
- Close the eyes and become conscious of whole body.
- Now get conscious of the inner self and relax mentally.
- Release all the tensions and get in complete harmony with the body.
- Get the conscious level to the sole of the feet.
- Let it go in the floor along with all the tensions as if by the gravity.
- Experience the surging vital force from the earth, enveloping the entire being.
- Finally raise the consciousness level between the eye brows.
- Envision the bright crimson sun flooding your entire being with its vibrant, vital and healing beams.
- Now get in the practice of all Suryanamaskarasana in one smooth synchronized go intertwined with another like a rhythmical dancing movement.

Contraindications
- Fever, acute inflammation, boils or rashes
- High blood pressure
- Coronary artery diseases
- Hernia
- Intestinal tuberculosis
- Severe back problems
- Slipped disc
- Sciatica
- Menstruation
- 2nd or 3rd trimester pregnancy

Benefits

- Stimulates and balances endocrine, circulatory, respiratory and digestive systems

PRANAYAMA - BREATHING TECHNIQUES FOR BEGINNERS

Yoga Breathing or Pranayama revitalizes the body, steadies the emotions and creates great clarity of mind. Before practicing the exercises, you should be sure that you understand how to breathe correctly and how to make full use of the diaphragm. In order to facilitate the flow of Prana and ensure that there is space for expanding the lungs, Yoga Breathing exercises are performed sitting down with the spine, neck and head in a straight line - either in the Easy Pose, the Lotus Pose or if neither is comfortable, sitting on a chair.

Beginner Yoga Breathing Techniques

Kapalabhati and Anuloma Viloma are of equal importance in the Basic Session of Asanas and should form the backbone of your Pranayama. Practice them exclusively to begin with, before your daily set of Asanas.

KAPALABHATI

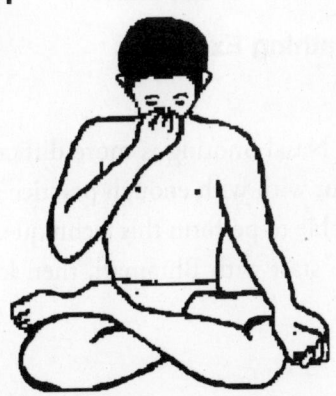

Fig. 1.5 – Kapalbhati

Kapalabhati is a Breathing Technique used specifically for cleansing. If you have a lot of mucus in the air passages or feel tension and blockages in the chest it is often helpful to breathe quickly. This article will introduce you to this breathing techniques and show you its its benefits.

ANULOM VILOM

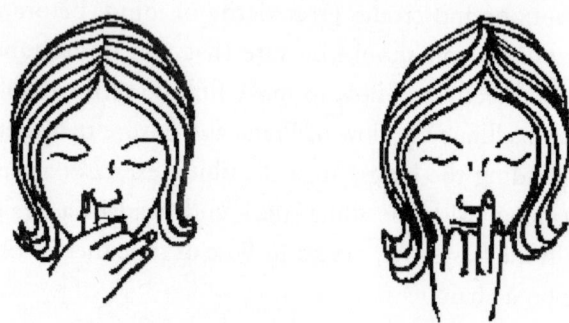

Fig. 1.6 – Alternate Nostril Breathing (Anulom Vilom)

Anuloma Viloma is also called the Alternate Nostril Breathing Technique. In this Breathing Technique, you inhale through one nostril, retain the breath, and exhale through the other nostril. Learn how to do this technique for beginners by following the steps found in this article.

Other Yoga Breathing Exercises

Bhramari

Bhramari or Nasal Snoring is more difficult than the usual mouth snoring. But with with enough practice and patience, you will eventually be able to perform this technique. If you are unsure where and how to start with Bhramari, then let this article help you.

Sitkari

Sitkari pertains to the sound made by drawing air in

through the front teeth-either tightly closed or slightly opened-with the tongue tip regulating the air pressure and sound. Learn more about this technique in this article.

Sithali

The breathing technique Sithali or tongue hissing refers to the sound caused when air is drawn in through the protruding tongue folded into a tube. This basic breathing technique can be performed by following the steps found in this article.

As already mentioned above, Pranayama revitalizes one's body along with other benefits that a person gets by practicing it. We hope that the different breathing techniques featured above will help you kick start your practice of Pranayama. But more than just encouraging you to practice Pranayama more, we also hope that with its help, you will be able to achieve the goals of performing it - to achieve balance in your life.

PADANGUSTHASANA

Sensitive people may have difficulty in expressing their emotions. According to psychologists, these feelings of frustration, anxiety or anger show up as a nasal symptoms. *Padangusthasana* is one of the asanas recommended for nasal symptoms and allergies.

Technique of Padangusthasana

- Pada means the foot Angustha are the big toes. This posture is attained by standing and holding the big toes.
- Stand in Tadasana
- Bring hands to the horizontal position and palms facing the floor
- Raise the hands vertically, above the head, palms facing forward biceps touching your ears.

- Slowly bend the back from base with hands parallel to the ground.
- Exhale, bend further forward and hold the big toes between the thumbs and the first two fingers, so that the palms face each other. Hold them tight.
- Keep the head up, stretch the diaphragm towards the chest and make the back as concave as possible. Instead of stretching down from the shoulders, bend forward from the pelvis.
- Keep the legs stiff and do not slacken the grip at the kness and toes. Stretch the shoulder blades also. Inspire once or twice in this position.
- Now exhale, and bring the head in between the knees by tightening the knees and pulling the toes without lifting them off the floor. Remain in this pose for about 20 seconds and maintaining normal breathing.
- Inhale, raise the head, release toes and stand up and return to *Tadasana*.

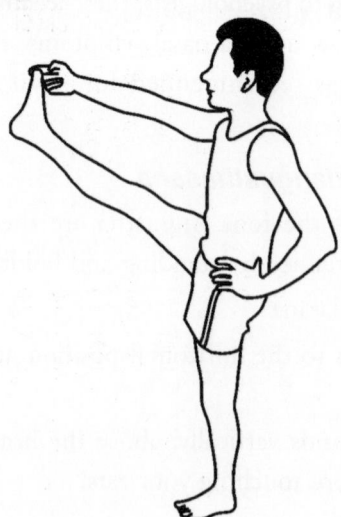

Fig. 1.7 – Padangusthasana

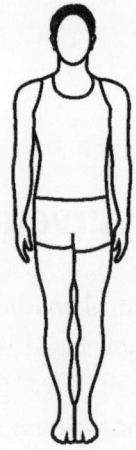

Fig. 1.7 – Tadasana

REFERENCES

1. http://yogaholidays.net/magazine/jalaneti.htm
2. http://www.healthandyoga.com/htm/clean/nasal.html
3. http://www.healthlibray.com/reading/ncure/nacure/tablexi.html
4. http://www.deccanherald.com/deccanherald.com/deccanherald/july092004/liv7.asp

CHAPTER 27

Ayurveda

Ayurveda is the traditional holistic medical system originated in India, using a constitution based model for determining the state of health. Thousands of years ago, Indian *rishis* and *seers* observed the rhythms of the universe and the interaction of the flow of energy throughout the body/mind during deep states of meditation — these insights form the basis of *Ayurveda, the "Science of Life"*, and were documented in ancient Indian tests such as the *Charaka Samhita*.

Ayurveda describes three fundamental body types or **doshas**, called **Vata**, **Pitta** and **Kapha**, which embody different combinations of the five elements: Air, Ether, Fire, Water and Earth. Each person contains all doshas in varying degrees, and their balance can be determined through examination of eyes, nails, tongue, skin voice, by pulse diagnosis, and through the insight of the ayurvedic practitioner. Because the five elements exist in the body and also in nature, the *doshas* can become aggravated or imbalanced due to inappropriate or inadequate diet, change of seasons and environmental factors etc. and therefore result in dissuasive diseases of the body. Ayurveda also describes three primary qualities of Nature, or **gunas**, called **Sattva** (equilibrium, evolution, intelligence), **Rajas** (activity, agitation) and **Tames** (inertia). These inner qualities are essential for the creation of all things in the material universe. They are sometimes referred to as the *"mental doshas"* as they describe the qualities and activities of the mind. Living in society requires a balance between *Sattva, Rajas and Tamas* — an imbalance can result in a restless, agitated or dull mind and disturbs the balance of Vata, Pitta and Kapha, leading to various ailments.

Ayurveda's focus on an individual's holistic health rather than merely the physical body, is the most beneficial aspect of ayurvedic medicine. It works on the principle that a perfect health condition is achievable through the psychosomatic integration in a person. Ayurveda provides us with a unique physical purification method called *panchakarma* and various ayurvedic herbal health remedies for mental and spiritual well-being.

The ultimate goal of ayurveda is to create a state of holistic health for the individual, to create, consequently, a healthy society and environment with its herbal health remedies. To attain this state ayurveda believes one's life must move in harmony with nature's rhythms and its laws. Because, ayurvedic medicine recognizes the human body is part of nature, rather a microcosm of the universe. The five great elements of the universe forms the three *doshas* of the human body, and a balance among the three *doshas* is necessary for the perfect working of the whole mechanism of body, mind and soul.

These holistic health benefits of ayurveda encompasses the physical, mental as well as the spiritual aspects of a person.

PHYSICAL BENEFITS

According to ayurveda each individual is a combination of the three *doshas* of *vata*, *pitta* and *kapha* or one of these *doshas*. The basic constitution represents the individual's psychological and physical nature, distinctly. The *tridoshas* governs all metabolic activities in an individual. Within each person the *doshas* are adjusting to countless changes in the *doshas* of nature, in addition to the changes within one self.

Noninvasive diagnostic ayurvedic treatments are beneficial for chronic patients suffering from diseases such as diabetes, heart ailments and cancer. Ayurvedic medicine resorts to outward diagnosis of symptoms by studying a patients' habits—diet and daily life, pulse, tongue, nail, face, lip, eye, nature of perspiration etc. Difficult diseases like asthma and tumor growths (*gulmas*) are managed effectively by these diagnostic methods.

Detoxification methods of ayurveda like *panchakarma* and other herbal health remedies, when applied wholly or singly, make the body more responsive to medicines and treatment. It hastens the healing process.

Various *yogasanas* prescribed by ayurveda help prevent the diseases from occuring and accumulating. *Yogasanas* achieve the twin purpose of strengthening body-parts such as bones, muscle and vital organs like heart, liver, stomach, intestine as well as keeping our blood circulation and psychological conditions strong and resilient.

Most importantly, a discerning diet according to one's *dosha* type, and well-regulated life (*dinacharya*) helps strengthen one's natural immune system.

PSYCHOLOGICAL BENEFITS

Perhaps ayurveda is the first such medical systems who recognizes that all diseases are but the direct manifestation of one's mental conditions. It says human mind consists three states or *trigunas*—*sattva*, *rajas* and *tamas*. Any disturbances in the equilibrium of the *tri-gunas*, manifest in physical illness according to the intensity or nature of the disturbances. In fact, the condition of body and mind are integral to the overall health of an individual.

When the mind is stressed the stress hormone cortisone is released by adrenal glands. The level of hormone released affects the total volume of the brain's hippocampus, which regulates our memory. Stress also affects all our decision-making activities in every field of life. Ayurveda stresses on four principles—regulation in *ahara* (food habit), *vihara* (activities), *nidra* (sleeping habit), and *maithuna* (sexual habit), to maintain the balance and equanimity of the mind. Especially its guidelines for an intelligently regulated diet and daily routine are, now, accepted techniques for stress management.

Ayurvedic massages, inhalation of herbal (Aromatherapy) preparations, *panchakarma* (*nasya*) besides the much-tested *yogasanas* and meditation leave a calming effect on the nerves.

According to ayurveda, *tamasic* (inertia, short of judgment) and *rajasic* (excessive activities, short of judgment) tendencies of mind prompt an individual to indulge in criminal or violent activities, telling lies and other such misconduct. This gives rise to negative thoughts like fear, anxieties, insecure feeling, greed, jealousy and anger.

SPIRITUAL BENEFITS

Various advanced ayurvedic treatments were born out of a necessity to keep the mind and body in perfect shapes to pursue the path of self-realization. Each individual is believed to possess undefined measures of creative capability, which, ideally, need to be realized. To achieve this, ayurveda emphasizes that the individual has to experience its oneness with the universe. The balance of *tri-doshas* and *tri-gunas* is imperative in this regard, for the individual needs to remain in balance within itself and in harmony outside with the nature.

The treatment methods, diet and lifestyle regimen in ayurveda are meticulously planned to heal the body as well as enrich the mind and the soul of each different individual. So that each can improve from their own levels to the higher goal of realizing the full self-potential. It was with ayurveda that the unique longevity and rejuvenating method of *rasayana* was born for mankind to progress in the path of spirituality.

Treatment

Rather than treating the symptoms of disease directly, ayurvedic treatment aims to repellence the doshas according to each person's constitution resulting in a body and mind that is healthy and sound. By becoming familiar with his/her unique *dosha* pattern, the patient can lead a life that is in harmony with individual's nature.

Panchakarma

The object of Panchakarma is to cleanse the human body and eliminate the various types of toxins that accumulate in the body. In ayuveda, these toxins are *ama (minute toxic matter)* and *malla (gross toxic matter)*. Panchakarma is helpful for both the healthy and the sick, and ideally a treatment course should be done once in a year. Prior to commencing this treatment, a consultation is required. Usually this treatment plan is completed within seven days period (,i e. two hours per day), depending on the patient's condition.

Ayurvedic Medications

Ayurvedic medicines and supplements are traditionally classified as being for *Vata, Pitta or Kapha* imbalances, hence often one type of preparation is able to treat many disorders. One example is medication for nasal problems such as sinusitis, which also works for digestion, influenza, headache, and general vitality. When Pitta is low then, Fire (*Agni*) is low, and toxic substances start to accumulate in different channels of the body due to low metabolic rate. This creates congestion in the flow of energy in the different channels. When this occurs, blockage of the mind, depression, anxiety and all sorts problems may result. *Guduchi*, for instance, is one of the ayurvedic herbs that can strengthen the immune system of the body. It has anti-inflammatory properties and is useful in treating upper respiratory disorders.

It may be noted that:

- According to ayurvedic principles a single herb may have an imbalancing or aggravating effect upon the *doshas*, and so, many herbs are combined together to counterbalance this factor. Many formulations contain ten, twenty or more types of herbs and minerals and are often ground for many hours over a period of days or months to increase their potency.
- The way in which the medication is ingested in also important. It is taken with an appropriate vehicle, (e.g. honey, warm milk, water and juice) which helps to provide the right therapeutic effect.
- Ayurveda also recommends *neti* cleansing is helpful for *Kapha* imbalances, which result in conditions such as nasal congestion, sinusitis, bronchial asthma, mental anxieties and other disorders.

REFERENCES

1. http://www.yatan-ayur.com.au/neti_post.htm
2. http://www.yatan-ayur.com.au/himalayan_herbal_mineral_remedies.htm

CHAPTER **28**

Naturopathy Combined With Yoga

Naturopathy is a natural healing technique using the healing powers of Nature. The principle of naturopathy is that the accumulation of toxins is the root cause of all diseases. Prevention and elimination of toxins is the route to health. Treatments are based on the five great elements of nature that have immense healing properties. There is no role of internal medication in the nature care system.

A sample regimen in naturopathy recommended for wide range of respiratory disorders such as rhinitis, sinusitis, nose block, nasal polyps and asthma etc. is as follows:

Common Programme

For all diseases as specified here under (for a required period):

1. Cold hip bath-evening for 15 minutes followed by brisk walk or yoga.
2. Mud pack-morning for 15/20 minutes, followed by neem (warm) water enema, if constipated/during fasting.
3. Oil massage for 30/40 minutes (once or twice a week).
4. Sauna/steam bath/sun bath (once or twice a week), if possible drink water before any hot treatment.
5. Relaxation, immersion-full bath (once or twice a week).

Specific Programme

1. Excent cold hip bath in common programme mentioned aboved, cold chest pack at night is given. Fomentation to upper back is beneficial.
2. *Thorough overhauling of the whole system* with fasting and enema for 3 to 8 days, dry friction, neutral sponge, breathing exercises, hot epsom salt bath.
3. Hot water should be sipped when required and dairy products are to be avoided.
4. Take steam inhalation, back massage, hot arm and hot foot bath (combined for 15 minutes).
5. At night, rub menthol on chest and throat and cover it with woollen muffler before sleeping. Keep chest warm by wearing sweater and muffler.
6. Do not expose to cold. Gargle with warm salt (saline) water 2/3 times daily.
7. Restrict (mucusless) diet for 3 to 6 weeks. Take fruits and juice rich in Vit C. No cooked food in the evenings.
8. **Yoga:** *Kunjal, Jaleti* followed by drop ghee in nostrils, *Vastra dhauti, Lagushankna prakashalana, Suryanamaskara, Bbhujangasana, Shalabhasana, Paschimottanasana, Kapal bharti Bhastrika,*

REFERENCES

1. http://soukya.com/homeopathy.html
2. http://www.emedicine.com/ent/topic402.htm

CHAPTER **29**

TCM - Traditional Chinese Medicine

Traditional Chinese Medicine has its origin in ancient Taoist philosophy which views a person as an energy system in which body and mind are unified, each influencing and balancing the other. Unlike allopathic medicine which usually attempts to isolate and separate a disease from a person, Chinese medicine emphasizes a holistic approach that treats the whole person. Many people have found Traditional Chinese methods of healing as excellent tools for maintaining optimum health and perventing illness.

The Basic Principle of Yin and Yang

The theory of Yin and Yang holds that all things have two opposite aspects. *Yin and Yang*, which are both opposite and at the same time *interdependent*. This is a universal law of the material world

The ancient Chinese used water and fire to symbolize Yin and Yang. Anything moving, hot bright and Hyperactive is Yang, and anything quiescent, cold, dim and hypoactive is Yin. The properties of these two are not absolute but relative. As a person changes, the *Yin and Yang components change* at a gradual rate. These two opposites are not stationary but in constant motion. Yin and Yang to terchange as well as balance each other.

The Application Yin and Yang in Chinese Medicine

Each organ has elements of Yin and Yang within. The

histological structures and nutrients are yin, and the functional activities are yang. Even though one organ may be predominantly Yin (or Yang) in nature, the balance of two is maintained in the whole healthy body because the sum total of them will be in a fluctuating balance. If a condition of prolonged excess or deficiency of either Yin or Yang occurs then disease results.

A Case

A male from Italy, 40 years old, 1.80 meter tall and 85 kilos in weight.

Major Complaint:

Severe headache, frequent and serious nasal problems every two weeks with much nasal discharge, stabbing pains in heart shortness or breath, occasional breath during sleep, shrinking cold pains of the stomach with along other problems for 15 years. He took treatment by western medicine intermittently in Italy, USA and other countries since 15 years and has not been relieved successfully. On January 18, 2004, he come to the TCM center (located in Huaihua city, China via Hong Kong and Guangzhou).

After Treatment

After 36 days of comprehensive treatment by herbal decoction, acupuncture, massage, cupping, and moxa, the following report is given:

"The chronic and complex condition of the patient has been greatly improved. The body is much stronger and could fight against the external wind efficiently. No headache, no nasal problem re-occurrence, no heart pains, obviously increased ability to take deep breaths, even the hair begins to grow, sleep good, appetite good, spirited less, So the general recovery is unexpectedly stable and satisfactor."

Acupuncture

The ancient Chinese believed that there is a universal life energy called *Chi* or *Qi* present in every living creature. This energy is said to circulate throughout the body along specific pathways that are called meridians. As long as this energy flows freely throughout the meridians, health is maintained, but once the flow of energy is blocked, the system is disrupted and pain and illness occur. Acupuncture works to "re-program" and restore normal functions by stimulating certain points on the meridians in order to free the *Chi* energy.

Treatment

A combination of acupuncture and Chinese herbs is often used to balance, unblock or strengthen the energy, depending on the patient's constitution and pathology, and herbs to strengthen the *Wei Qi* (this is the defensive energy that blocks out pathogens, i.e. irritants, pollen, bacteria and viruses etc.) If the symptoms have progressed from a runny nose to sticky yellow mucus with red, hot itchy and swollen eyes, it is believed in Chinese medicine that the pathology has gone from Wind-Cold to Wind-Heat. In such cases, other herbs are added which can clear heat and resolve phlegm/mucus.

It has been reported that this method is successful even with cases with a history of nasal problems for as long as 15 years. The underlying pathology is treated with acupuncture concentrating on making the Lung Qi descend to stop sneezing and breathing at the same time unblocking Liver Qi stangnation to relieve stress, combining both body and ear acupuncture. This is supplemented with herbal formulas (*Yu Ping Feng San*), containing only a few herbs. Good progress is observed within two weeks.

Tai chi

This is a gentle martial art that involves a combination of meditation and flowing exercises to help improve the health of the body and mind. *Tai Chi Chuan* means "Supreme Ultimate Boxing." The Supreme Ultimate here refers to the Tao, or more specifically, the framework within which the dualities of *Yin* and *Yang* manifest themselves in the field of time. The allusion to the Tai Chi in this context suggests that the art contains within itself (in its movements, shapes and patterns of breathing) all that is necessary for these dynamic forces to interact and to be reconciled.

Practice

Tai Chi Chuan is a practice of meditation within movement, a series of movements performed in a slow, relaxed and harmonised way. It is the *Taoist path* to mental, physical and spiritual well being as well as being a powerful 'internal' martial art. The gentle nature of Tai Chi Chuan makes it suitable for people of all ages and ability. Practicing *Tai Chi* can be a very pleasurable experience, one that unites body and mind which feel invigorated and refreshed.

Benefits of Tai Chi

- Daily practice of Tai Chi promotes mental clarity and a healthy body, assists with balance and help the cirulation of blood.
- Tai Chi has proven to improve lung elesticity, balance blood pressure and reduce the impact of ageing.
- With regular practice it can relive stress and *improve metabolism and the immune system.*
- A feeling of profound well being and mental calmness can result from regular practice.

REFERENCES

1. http://www.tcmtreatment.com/Giacomo.htm
2. http://www.acupuncture.com/conditions/hayfever.htm
3. http://www.devontaichi.co.uk/about_practice.php

CHAPTER **30**

Nutritional Supplements and Dietary Advice to Patients

ROLE OF DIET AND PROPER NUTRITION IN TREATMENT

Many diseases are directly or indirectly due to an inproper diet. If diet and habit are properly regulated, cure becomes easier and more smooth, hence regulation of diet is one of the most important prerequisites of homeopathic treatment. The role of diet and proper nutrition was first recognized by **Dr. Hahnemann**[1] who is known to have given a diet sheet along with the prescription to his patients in Paris. The importance of diet is also evident from the aphorisms 259 - 261 in the Organon, where he states, Breach "..... *as their diseases are aggravated by such noxious influences and other disease causing errors in diet and regimen, which often pass unnoticed*"

- Aphorism 260.

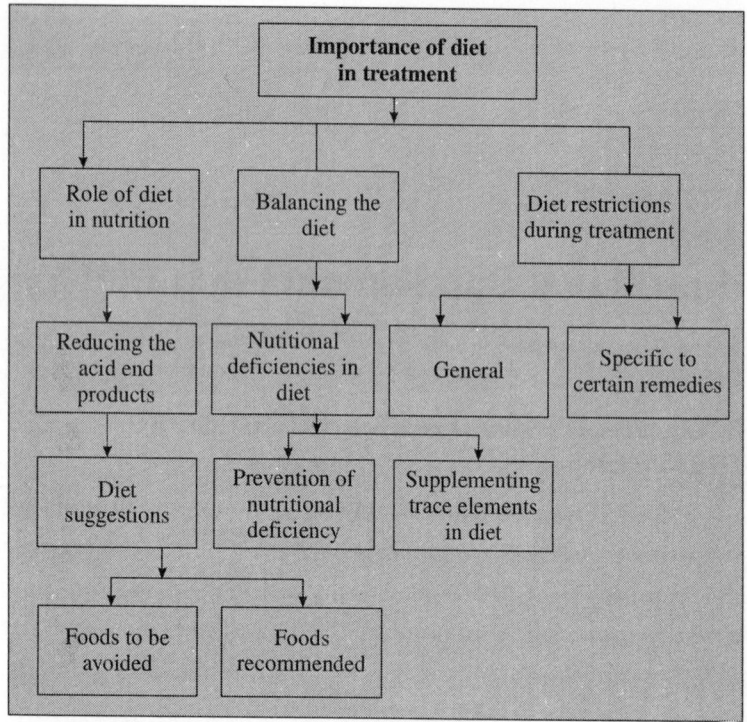

The importance of diet in treatment may be represented schematically in a flow-chart as above:

BALANCING THE DIET TO REDUCE ACID BREACH END-PRODUCTS

Patients may be advised to avoid acid forming foods like refined foods white flour and white sugar; as well as excess of protein foods such as meat, cheese and fish. "Anything that depletes the body's alkaline reserves depletes its functional activity....4/5th of the daily foods should therefore consist of the base-forming things such as *vegetable, raw salads* and *fresh fruits*", according to **Dr. Hay** in "A new Health Era" as quoted by **T S Iyer**[2] (*Beginner's Guide to Homoeopathy*)

PREVENTING NUTRITIONAL DEFICIENCIES IN DIET

The immune system is essential in warding off diseases and it requires minerals, vitamins and trace elements for proper functioning. Hence the *diet must be supplemented* to include the necessary *minerals, vitamins and trace elements* such as *Selenium, Copper, Cobalt, Manganese*, etc. More importantly, trace elements and vitamins work in corelation and *a balanced intake is necessary.*

SUPPLEMENTING TRACE ELEMENTS AND VITAMINS IN DIET

Dr. Fullerton believes that diet supplements may often help to avoid aggravations in homeopathic treatment. It may also be advisable to *take the supplements few days before starting the remedy,* so that there is a better response to homeopathic treatment. For instance, there was an aggravation with break *Hepar sulph.*, while treatment a cal, but after receiving *Zinc* supplements, the calf responded well to *Hepar sulph.*, without any aggravation.

It has been noted that an aggravation may be due to a deficiency that must be rectified before trying the remedy again. A palliative remedy may be tried in the meantime.

Pulsatilla is a constitutional remedy and it has been suggested that it is beneficial to supplement *Pulsatilla* therapy with *Vitamin B6 and E, Zinc, Magnesium* and *Selenium* to prevent aggravation.

SUGGESTIONS TO REPLACE UNDESIRABLE FOODS WITH RECOMMENDED FOODS

Foods to be Avoided or Minimized

Patients with rhinitis symptoms are advised to avoid food items which may trigger their symptoms such as sneezing. They may include cold drinks, certain fruits like citrus fruits, processed foods and certain spices. In general, it is advisable to refrain from or minimize the use of the following food items *while taking homeopathic treatment* since they reduce the efficacy of the homeopathic remedies.

Avoid or Minimize:
- Coffee (especially black coffee which can be anti-dotal)
- Strong tea
- Strong smelling food substances such as spices, camphor, ginger, asofetida, garlic, onion, mint, radish, pickles, etc.
- All refined or processed foods such as white sugar, white flour and white rice
- Milk products – Adult patients may be advised to reduce the quantity of milk products after a certain age since digestion becomes weaker with age

Recommended Foods
- In place of coffee or tea, drinks made from malt, ovaltine, oats porridge, butter milk, cereals, broken wheat or rice may be used. (Strong coffee or tea are stimulants and can bring about nervous depression and other disorders like dyspepsia, high blood pressure, etc.)
- Plenty of fresh vegetables and fruits (which are agreeable to the patient).
- *Unrefined sugars* like jaggery, brown sugar or honey have a better food value and may be used instead of white sugar, which can cause irritation in the stomach
- *For* rhinitis patients, processed foods could be a source of irritants or allergens. White flour and white rice may be substituled with unrefined wholemeal flour, *handpounded* rice and other whole grains which contain more fibre and help to avoid constipation.

- According to T S Iyer[2], milk should be taken slowly and in small quantities only

DIET RESTRICTIONS DURING TREATMENT

It is important that food taken is light, easy to digest, nutritive and is in just enough quantity to satisfy hunger. If the patients suffer from the following disorders, in addition to rhinitis, they *have to be informed or reminded* about the following important guidelines for diet while treating these disorders:s

- *Diabetics* : Avoid-sweet fruits, sugar, synthetic sweeteners like saccharin, potatoes, and starchy vegetables

    Milk in limited quantites, butter milk, vegetables

- *Dyspepsia* : Avoid – fried food in fat or oils, milk products, white sugar and white flour. Allowed - Boiled or steamed vegetables, butter milk instead of milk

- *Constipation* : Avoid or reduce the use of purgative and laxatives, Allowed : Take diet rich in fibres such as vegetables and fruits like figs, prunes and dates. Drink plenty of water

- *Skin diseases* : Avoid – Sea food, shell fish, chillies, brinjals and too much sweets. Allowed-Use pepper instead of chillies

- *Diarrhea* : Reduce the intake of milk

    Allowed – Take light porridge and butter milk

- *High blood pressure* : Avoid – Tea, coffee, condiments. Reduce the intake of salt

- *Liver disorders* : Reduce the intake of alcohol, tea and coffee. Avoid high protein foods and also fats like cream. Allowed – Take greens and fresh vegetables.

- *Chronic rheumatism* : Eat less in general. Avoid – or reduce the intake of meat.

- **Dr. J B D' Castro** recommends asparagus in diet, as it is excellent for rheumatism.
- *Kidney disorders :* Avoid - Excess protein in foods, salt and condiments, tea, coffee and eggs. Allowed - Barley, butter milk, low protein foods.
- *Cancer* : Avoid-Meat and fleshy foods of all types. Allowed - Take more greens and fresh vegetables.
- *Asthma :* Avoid - Tea, coffee, watery vegetables or fruits to which the patient is sensitized.

Foods to be Avoided While Taking Homeopathic Remedies

Sometimes, certain specific substances need to be avoided with some medicines. For example, **Dr J.B.D. Castro** suggests the following in *"What a Homeopath Should Know Before Prescribing?"*

- *Natrium mur* – While taking Nat-m., menthol or peppermint is to be avoided
- *Sulphur* – With Sulphur, it is better not to take chamomile tea
- *Sepia* – When Sepia is given, it is advisable to stop vinegar and lemon or anything sour
- *Lycopodium* – With Lycopodium, oysters may be avoided

Bibliography:

1. Samuel Hahnemann; 2003; *Organon of Medicine,* Reprint Ed.; B. Jain Publishers, New Delhi
2. T S Iyer; 2004; *Beginner's Guide to Homeopathy,* Reprint Ed.; B. Jain Publishers, New Delhi
3. The British Institute of Homeopathy - Postgrauate course; B. Jain Publishers, New Delhi
4. J B D' Castro; 2000; *What a Homeopath Should Know Before Prescribing,* Reprint Ed. B. Jain Publishers

CHAPTER **31**

Conclusion - Living with Rhinitis

With your best endeavor you will make mistakes, but make them as few as you can.

J. T. Kent *(Lesser Writings)*

To summarise, there are two basic types of rhinitis – allergic rhinitis and non-allergic rhinitis (the most common type of which is called vasomotor rhinitis). Symptoms of non-allergic rhinitis may resemble those of allergic rhinitis – A chronic running nose, sneezing episodes, lachrymation, itching in nose or mouth, nasal drainage and nasal congestion. The treatment, however, is similar to allergic rhinitis – mainly avoidance and medication.

Short Term Relief

The commonly used treatment options for rhinitis in conventional medicine are anti-histamine nose sprays, anti-histamine tablets, and anti-inflammatory glucocorticosteroid nosal sprays-all of which have their side effects. A lot of rhinitis sufferers got relief from decongestants taken orally. Some people may suffer such a severe onset of the problem that they need *cortisone* drugs applied to the nasal membranes. Over-the-counter decongestant nasal sprays may give temporary relief, but it is usually quite short-lived and they can, with excessive use, rebound swelling worse than the original probelm. It is better to try and get along without without them.

Long Term Solution - Homeopathy

As has been discussed in this pater, a holistic approach, integrating the man and his mind, is advisable to cope with the problem in the long term. Here the advantages of homeopathy as an alternative therapy are obvious. Homeopathy not only heals the body, but treats the patient as a whole, giving equal importance to his mental and emotional symptoms.

A literature search covering books, journals as well as web sites, reveals that not enough attention has been paid to this problem and it would be profitable to do a more comprehensive research in this area. Homeopathy offers a holistic treatment, but a complete cure may still be elusive although a *successful management* of the case is very much possible, as evident from the case studies reported earlier.

The fact remains that persistent rhinitis is an ongoing (chronic) condition that needs regular treatment to prevent or minimize symptoms. Rhinitis may seem simple, but, being 'multimiasmatic', it is very difficult to cure. However, with homeopathic treatment over a period of time, the condition eases and becomes manageable without the aid of conventional medications, affording great relief to the long-suffering patients.

"In this life, we can not do great things. We can only do small things with great love."

– **Mother Teresa**

Bibliography

Bibliography and references have been given *at the end of each chapter.* Following are the main sources of reference

Books :
1. Allen, H C; Allen's Keynotes - Rearranged and Classified, Reprint Ed.; B. Jain Publishers, New Delhi.
2. Banerjea, S K; *Miasmatic Diagnosis,* Reprint Ed.; B. Jain Publishers, New Delhi.
3. Bishambar Das, R; Select Your Remedy, Revised Ed.; Bishambar Free Homeo Dispensary, New Delhi.
4. Boericke, William; Homeopathic Materia Medica and Repertory, Reprint Ed.; B. Jain Publishers, New Delhi.
5. Farrington, E A; *Comparative Materia Medica,* Reprint Ed.; B. Jain Publishers, New Delhi.
6. Gunavante, S M; *The Genius of Homeopathic Remedies,* Reprint Ed.; B. Jain Publishers, New Delhi.
7. Gunavante, S M; *Introduction to Homeopathic Prescribing,* Reprint Ed.; B Jain Publishers, New Delhi.
8. Gupta, R L; *Unique Compilations with Clinical Cases in Homeopathy and Biochemic,* Reprint Ed.; B. Jain Publishers, New Delhi.
9. Gupta, S C; *What if a Well Selected Remedy Fails in Homeopathy,* Revised Ed.; B. Jain Publishers, New Delhi.

10. Hahnemann, Samuel; *Organon of Medicine,* Reprint Ed.; B. Jain Publishers, New Delhi.
11. Iyer, T S; *Beginner's Guide to Homeopathy,* Reprint Ed.; B Jain Publishers, New Delhi.
12. Jayasuria, Anton; *A to Z Homeopathy,* Reprint Ed.; B. Jain Publishers, New Delhi.
13. Kent, James Tyler, *Lectures on Homeopathic Materia Medica,* Reprint Ed.; B. Jain Publishers, New Delhi.
15. Kinra, Ritu; *Materia Medica of Students,* Reprint Ed.; B. Jain Publishers, New Delhi.
16. Nash, E B; *Leaders in Homeopathic Therapeutics,* Reprint Ed.; B. Jain Publishers, New Delhi.
17. Rowe, Todd; *Homeopathic Methodology - Repertory, Case Taking and Case Analysis*
18. Siva Shankar, K; 1995; *Homeopathy for Every Family,* First Ed.; Shanti Homeo Stores, Hyderabed.
19. Thombre, P B; 2002; *Gems of Organon,* Reprint Ed.; B. Jain Publishers, New Delhi.
20. Uniyal, Pameeta; 2005; *Materia Medica for Students,* First Ed.; B Jain Publishers, New Delhi.
21. Vithoulkas, George; 2004; *The Science of Homeopathy,* Reprint Ed.; B. Jain Publishers, New Delhi.
22. Vithoulkas, George; 2004; *The Science of Homeopathy,* Reprint Ed.; B. Jain Publishers, New Delhi.
23. 'The British Institute of Homeopathy - *Post-graduate course';* B. Jain Publishers, New Delhi.

Websites:

i. http://www.homeoint.org;

ii. http://www.mayoclinic.com/health

Appendix - A General Questionnaire Designed for Rhinitis Patients

MEDICAL AND PERSONAL HISTORY

To determine the cause of rhinitis, the patient needs to be asked the following questions:

- The time of day and time of year of occurence of rhinitis episodes. The timing of symptoms or whether they are persistent throughout the year, helps to determine if the problem is one of seasonal allergies.
- If there is a history of medical problems
- In women, whether they are pregnant or taking estrogen containing agents (oral contraceptives, hormone replacement therapy)
- If the patient is taking any other medications, including on-going decongestants (*which could be causing a rebound effect*).
- *Any additional unusual symptoms.* For example:
  - Bloody nasal discharge and obstruction in only one nasal passage could suggest a tumor
  - Swelling or tingling of the lips after eating raw stoned-fruit may indicate seasonal allergies
  - Fatigue, sensitivity to cold, weight gain and depression may be signs of hypothyroidism

- Rhinitis that appears seasonally is almost always due to pollens and outdoor allergens
- If symptoms occur throughout the year, perennial allergic or non-allergic rhinitis may be suspected

The questionnaire below is a sample format and may be used in clinics to check the type of rhinitis that a particular individual suffers from.

A knowledge of trigger factors for rhinitis is useful in order to avoid or minimize exposure to the "maintaining cause" in future. A history of the past medications is also useful to know, especially to rule out drug-induced rhinitis

RHINITIS SCREENER

Instructions to the Patient : Please Complete the Checklist

1. Do you experience any of these symptoms?

Symptom	Mild	Moderate	Severe
Stuffy nose	☐	☐	☐
Sneezing	☐	☐	☐
Running nose	☐	☐	☐
Itchy nose	☐	☐	☐
Post-nasal drip	☐	☐	☐
Watery eyes	☐	☐	☐
Itchy eyes, ears, or throat	☐	☐	☐

2. When do you experience these symptoms?
(Check all that apply)

☐ In the spring
☐ In the summer
☐ In the winter

☐ In the fall
☐ All year long

3. Which irritants or allergens make your symptoms worse? *(Check all that apply)*

Allergic cause	*Non-allergic cause*
☐ Grass	☐ Cigarette smoke
☐ Hat	☐ Perfumes
☐ Pollen	☐ Exhaust fumes (cars)
☐ Dust	☐ Cold days
☐ Mould	☐ Temperature changes
☐ Pets	☐ Alcohol (beer, wine)

Others (please indicate)

4. Which medications have you used so far? *(Check all that apply)*

Anti-histamines	*Past*	*Present*
Allegra	☐	☐
Astelin	☐	☐
Clarinex	☐	☐
Claritin	☐	☐
Zyrtec	☐	☐
Nasal corticosteroids	☐	☐
Flonase	☐	☐
Nasonex	☐	☐
Rhinocort	☐	☐
Vancenase@ AB	☐	☐

Other (please indicate)

Source:

http://www.astelin.com/rhinitisproblem/screener.html